DEDICATION

To friends and family who faithfully cheer us on, to our mentors and coaches, to our buddies, and most of all to God....Thank you.

ISBN: 978-0-6151-8291-9

Go to any bookstore, and you will see numerous self-improvement and fitness books. The workout market is massive in today's society. Everywhere you turn, there are overweight people searching for a magic potion that will help them lose weight. As a physician, nearly every day I encounter someone asking for a way to lose weight. I am repeatedly giving the common medical advice of exercising and losing weight to combat obesity related diseases including diabetes, high cholesterol, and coronary artery disease. However, there are no magic pills. It takes hard work and discipline to be successful at weight loss and to stay in shape. The excuses for not doing so are many: "I'm too busy", "It's too boring", "I can't afford a gym membership or expensive workout equipment", etc., etc

In this manual, we present a program to blow all of these excuses away. The exercise routines are exciting, simplified, quick, and effective. But why should you read this manual? The reason is that no other fitness approach comes from such a varied background of military Special Forces, collegiate, and professional training. All of this information is grounded in the fact that a medical doctor has developed it and proven its results!

The MAXimize the MINimum workout is designed to be adaptable for all levels of motivation and fitness ability. The one common denominator in the athletes experiencing success on this program is that they are all busy people unable to spend hours every day at the gym. Start out slowly or take it to the max right away. It's up to you.

-Dr. BIG WIG

REVIEWERS:

Karrn E. Gustafson, DO
Captain USAF
Family Practice Physician
Mountain Home AFB, Idaho
Ironman triathlete, marathoner

Michael A. Howard, MD
Northwestern University Feinberg School of
Medicine
Plastic Surgeon
Chicago, Illinois
Ironman triathlete, marathoner

Michael M. Karch, MD
Mammoth Lakes Medical Group
Orthopaedic Surgeon

Maristela L. Onozato, MD, Ph.D.
Georgetown University Medical Center
Washington, D.C.

Mammoth Lakes, California
*Ultramarathoner, Ironman triathlete,
marathoner*

Benjamin E. Hubbert
SSgt USAF
Instructor Combat Control Orientation Course
San Antonio, Texas
Triathlete

Greg J. Hericks
MSgt USAF
Superintendent Combat Control Orientation
Course
San Antonio, Texas
Triathlete

PREFACE

By alternating major muscle groups in a **timed** workout, the goal of this book is to **maximize both strength and endurance in a minimum amount of time (i.e., MAX the MIN)**. These workouts are designed not only for people who want to improve their physical fitness and have limited time and resources, but for serious athletes who want to improve their performance in any particular sport of interest. Instructive photographs will facilitate learning the proper form and techniques. The only equipment you will need is access to a pullup/dip bar. In addition to gyms, many parks and recreation areas will have this equipment. This equipment is also available over the internet or at your neighborhood sporting goods store at minimal cost.

You can start at whatever level fits into your lifestyle and baseline fitness level. For example, if you are not used to challenging routines, start at a beginner's level. If you are currently engaged in rigorous workouts as a professional, college, or high school athlete, start at a higher level of difficulty. Over time, the level of difficulty and repetitions increase. Some weeks are set aside for performance tests in order to monitor your progress. Other weeks are easier and designed as rest weeks. After approximately two weeks of doing the routines as described, you will notice improved strength and conditioning. After six weeks, you will see a significant improvement in your physical form. These workouts are not meant to be easy, but with them you will re-establish your physical limits. Stick to it, and you will see dramatic results.

James Bales, MD
Peter Andrews, PhD

INJURY DISCLAIMER

The authors and publisher of MAXimize the MINimum do not hold any liability, personal or professional, for injuries resulting from the misapplication of any of the training procedures described in this publication. One should always consult with a physician before beginning a rigorous exercise program, especially if any of the following risk factors are present: cardiovascular disease including chest pains at rest or exertion, family history of coronary heart disease before the age of 55, high cholesterol, cardiac arrhythmias, smoking, chronic hypertension, extreme obesity, chronic muscular or joint problems, pregnancy or within 3 months post-partum, recent surgery, arthritis, diabetes, asthma, or years of a sedentary lifestyle.

CONTENTS

Page Number

INTRODUCTION 2

CHAPTER 1: How & Why I Get Health Benefits From This Workout? 4
(What physical exercise can do for you)

CHAPTER 2: How Do I Begin? 9
(The building blocks of success)

CHAPTER 3: Why Does Form Matter? 20
(Train how you want to look)

CHAPTER 4: The Routines 51
(Reaching your goal in the MIN amount of time)

CHAPTER 5: How Should I Eat To Perform At My Best? 64
(Using nutrition to your advantage)

CHAPTER 6: What Does Heart Rate Have To Do With Peak Performance? 79
(Exercise with your heart, not your legs)

CHAPTER 7: What About When I'm Traveling? 84
(Modified workouts for those on the road)

APPENDIX A: Weekly Schedules 86

APPENDIX B: Daily Training Log 88

APPENDIX C: Daily Nutrition Log 89

APPENDIX D: Monthly Training Log 90

REFERENCES 91

ABOUT THE AUTHORS 94

Front Cover: Dr. James R.T. Bales
Back Cover: Dr. Peter M. Andrews & Chan Lang

INTRODUCTION

Unless you are a professional athlete, you probably have a limited amount of time to exercise. You may strive for fitness, but with work, family, and other commitments, this seems difficult or almost impossible. In addition, most workouts are not balanced, but are focused on either aerobic (i.e. cardiovascular training) or anaerobic (i.e. weight lifting) exercise programs. Just go to the local gym and you will see the segregated areas. The anaerobic weight lifters never venture far from the weights, and the aerobic runners rarely stray from the elliptical machines, stationary bikes, and treadmills.

The routines described herein will, on the other hand, provide a combined aerobic and anaerobic workout *in a time efficient manner*. These routines do not incorporate weights, pulleys or complex equipment other than simple pullup and dip bars. They utilize your own body weight, working to increase muscle strength, coordination and endurance. By increasing coordination and strength through the resistance of your own body weight in multiple exercises, these workouts hope to reduce the chance of injury to any one area of your body.

Being able to push, pull and otherwise negotiate your own body results in strengthening and trimming effects that are difficult to obtain by solely working out with weights or solely performing aerobic activity. A total body workout is achieved by alternating major muscle groups and their associated stabilizing muscles. The human body will adopt a physical appearance in response to the demands placed on it. These routines will result in a considerable amount of body sculpting and loss of body fat.

As mentioned, an advantage to utilizing your own body weight is development of the stabilizing/finer muscle groups responsible for balance and coordination, while at the same time increasing lean muscle mass in the major muscle groups. Finally, because the routines are performed in a limited time period with an elevated heart rate, they result in an aerobic workout as well. For instance, running, swimming, and biking will result in considerable cardiovascular conditioning and muscle firming, but will not provide the upper body strength and muscle definition obtained from lifting weights. Lifting weights, on the other hand, is usually focused on providing muscle bulk, but provides less cardiovascular training.

The workouts set forth in this book are not easy. The more difficult will challenge professional athletes in both strength and endurance. At the same time, they will allow achievement of maximum performance in a minimum amount of time. This is an important concept because most individuals have aspects of their lives that are pulling them in different directions, making it difficult to maintain a regimented training plan.

As with many plans in life, many individuals enthusiastically begin a workout program, maintain it for a short while, but then falter requiring another start at square one. Others simply consider a workout program as too difficult, perhaps nearly impossible, and therefore never get started. Another trap that many succumb to is believing that they do not have the energy, time, or knowledge/ability for an effective workout within the time limitations they have. Finally, some believe that they need other individuals (e.g. personal trainer), to encourage them to succeed in a workout program. If you fall into any of the foregoing categories, the time efficient routines described herein are for you. As is often said, a healthy mind and healthy body go hand-in-hand. Feeling good and looking good provide encouragement as well as confidence and respect that will carry over to all aspects of your life. Do not rely on others to motivate you. Motivation has to come from within. Get started as soon as you have some free time that you might otherwise spend reading, watching TV, or engaging in conversation. Once you realize the benefits of these routines, you will become self-motivated and will succeed despite everyday obstacles and excuses.

2

Yes, You Can Do It All: Because the routines are time limited, you can continue to be actively involved in the other necessary and important facets of your life, yet maintain an effective workout program. The routines set forth in this book focus on strengthening every aspect of the body's musculature that is essential, not only for physical fitness performance, but for everyday living and health. Instead of isolating individual muscles, these exercises shift the focus on to the whole body working in unison. As a result, you will strengthen those core stabilizing muscles that are critical for everyday tasks. The core conditioning found in these workouts will give you coordinated body strength.

The routines described in this publication can be done nearly anywhere you can set up or have access to pullup/dip bars. They are time tested, built around exercise programs known to improve strength, fitness, flexibility and endurance.

Variations of these routines are used to train advanced armed services personnel as well as college, high school and professional athletes. They are designed to challenge the most advanced athlete as well as the beginner. In addition to the routines themselves, we have included a variety of ancillary concepts that will help to maximize your performance.

At its core is a philosophy that: you desire physical fitness and want to get the most out of your time and energy. This books' greatest contribution to you is: <u>Experience</u> - from people just like you who are maintaining fitness, <u>Honesty</u> - about what works and what doesn't, and <u>Perspective</u> – about how to juggle family, work, training and most importantly: life.

CHAPTER 1: How & Why I Get Health Benefits From This Workout?
(What physical exercise can do for you)

A wise man should consider that health is the greatest of human blessings…
-Hippocrates

In this chapter, we simply reiterate what most people already know: That exercise is good for your health and is an effective means of preventive medicine. If you are already convinced that this is true, you may skip this chapter, If not, read on.

It is therefore hard to understand why so few people regularly participate in an exercise program. According to the U.S. Surgeon General, more than 60 percent of adults in the United States do not engage in the recommended amount of activity, and approximately 25 percent of U.S. adults are not active at all. Most of those who do exercise are walkers and joggers, leaving a small percentage that workout in a well-balanced exercise program.

What this program can do for your physical health: While learning the facts, we can dispel some common misconceptions. Let's take a look at some of the health related reasons why we should engage in activities combining strength and endurance in a workout program.

- ***Avoid Metabolic Rate Reduction:*** Because muscle is very active tissue, muscle loss is accompanied by a reduction in our resting metabolism. The average adult experiences a 2-5 percent reduction in metabolic rate every decade of life. Some of this metabolic rate reduction is due to muscle loss; some is due to a slower paced lifestyle; and finally some is a natural part of aging. It has been estimated that a resting pound of adipose tissue (fat) requires approximately 2 kcal/hr for maintenance. On the other hand, a resting pound of lean muscle mass requires on the order of 35-50 kcal/hr. The calories or "fuel" consumed for maintenance of resting muscle should account for the majority of calories we should consume in a day. Thus, the more lean muscle mass you have, the higher your metabolic rate will be and the more food you will need to eat. The MAX the MIN workout incorporates strength exercises to prevent muscle loss and build lean muscle. In addition, it has an endurance component that will burn more calories per workout than strength training alone. The advantage of an elevated heart rate means that your metabolism will be revved up throughout your workout and will continue to burn at an increased rate for several hours after you finish.

- ***Increase Metabolic Rate:*** Research reveals that adding 3 pounds of muscle increases our resting metabolic rate by 7 percent and our daily calorie requirements by 15 percent. At rest, a pound of muscle requires about 35-50 calories per day for tissue maintenance, and during exercise muscle energy utilization increases dramatically. Adults with increased lean muscle mass use more calories all day long.

- ***Avoid Muscle and Bone Loss:*** After the early twenties, it has been estimated that adults who do not do some type of exercise or strength training routine lose between 5-7 pounds of muscle every decade. Simply walking or jogging regularly can improve cardiovascular fitness. However, it is not as efficient at preventing the loss of lean muscle or bone, especially in the upper extremities, as is an integrated strength/aerobic training program. As we age, the decrease in lean muscle and bone strength becomes increasingly important. By the time we reach our fifties, we are at increased risks for muscle strains and tears and fractures from falls due to this atrophy of muscle and bone. Osteoporosis is considered one to the greatest risks to the elderly, specifically women. An integrated program of strength and endurance exercises will help maintain muscle mass and bone strength throughout life.

- ***Increase Muscle:*** Physical activity will actively build lean muscle mass. While response to every workout program is slightly variable for different people, most will see changes in their bodies within 6 weeks. Athletes who begin at a higher level may not see as dramatic results as others who begin the MAX the MIN from a more sedentary lifestyle. Still, a basic principle of human physiology is that cells respond to stress. By increasing the physical stresses on your body through a program of combined strength and endurance training, your body will respond with stronger ligaments and tendons as well as with increased lean muscle mass.

- ***Increase Bone Density:*** The effects of exercise are similar for bone as well as muscle tissue. Repetitively loading our musculoskeletal system not only stimulates muscle hypertrophy, but also increases bone density. This decreases the risk for osteoporosis and the morbidity and mortality that goes with it in the form of hip fractures and spinal compression fractures.

- ***Reduce Body Fat:*** Obesity has been linked to many causes of death. The number one cause of death in the developed world continues to be heart disease, and obesity plays a major role. In addition, obesity has been linked to numerous types of cancers (including cancers of the breast (post-menopause), colon, endometrium, kidney, gallbladder, pancreas, ovaries, stomach and esophagus, fibromyalgia, fatigue, joint pain, sleep apnea, type 2 diabetes, high cholesterol, and high blood pressure. By decreasing your body fat you are actively making an effort to decrease these risks.

  - People who are obese have an abnormally high and unhealthy proportion of body fat. To measure obesity, researchers commonly use a formula based on weight and height known as the body mass index (BMI). BMI is the ratio of weight (in kilograms) to height (in meters) squared. BMI provides a more accurate measure of obesity or being overweight than does weight alone.
  - Guidelines established by the National Institutes of Health (NIH) place adults age 20 and older into one of four categories based on their BMI:

<18.5   underweight

18.5 to 24.9 Healthy

25.0 to 29.9 overweight

>30.0   Obese

The following chart can be used to determine BMI category. (Find the height, and move across the chart to the appropriate weight.)

Body Mass Index Chart, Adults 20 and Over

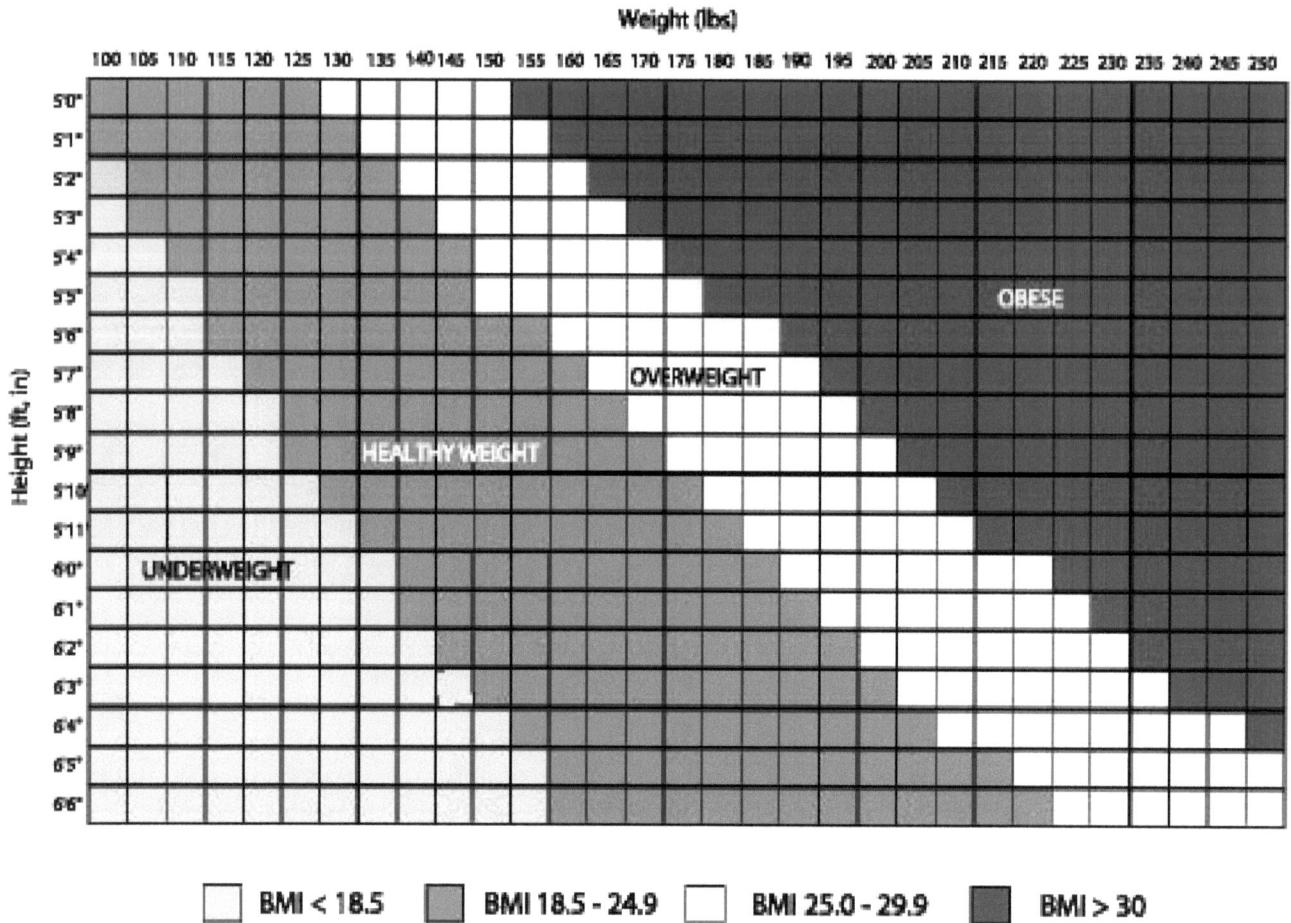

Weight (lbs)

A chart showing Height (ft, in) on the vertical axis from 5'0" to 6'6" and Weight (lbs) on the horizontal axis from 100 to 250. Labels within the chart read UNDERWEIGHT, HEALTHY WEIGHT, OVERWEIGHT, and OBESE.

Legend:
□ BMI < 18.5   ▨ BMI 18.5 - 24.9   □ BMI 25.0 - 29.9   ■ BMI > 30

- ***Improve Blood Lipid Levels:*** Another risk factor for heart disease and stroke is a high LDL cholesterol level (bad cholesterol), high triglycerides, and a low HDL cholesterol level (good cholesterol). Exercise has been found to lower LDL cholesterol and triglyceride levels, while at the same time increasing HDL cholesterol levels.

- ***Improve Glucose Metabolism:*** Resistance to glucose metabolism is associated with adult onset or Type 2 diabetes and associated with high levels of blood glucose. Glucose uptake is significantly increased in people who exercise. This is because working muscle burns glucose. People who workout have decreased problems with insulin resistance. Exercise combined with weight loss will lower blood glucose levels preventing or even potentially 'curing' adult onset diabetes.

- ***Increase Gastrointestinal Transit Time:*** Delayed gastrointestinal transit time is related to a higher risk of colon cancer. It has also been linked to constipation, therefore potentially leading to diverticulosis and diverticulitis. Therefore, an exercise program speeds up the gastrointestinal transit time, decreasing your risk of gastrointestinal problems.

- ***Reduce Resting Blood Pressure:*** High blood pressure, or hypertension, is one of the primary risk factors for stroke and heart failure. Exercise can reduce high blood pressure or decrease the risk of developing high blood pressure, therefore preventing the need to be on daily blood pressure medication.

- ***Reduce Low Back Pain:*** Strong low-back muscles are more likely to prevent back pain than weak back muscles. In people younger than 45 years old, mechanical low back pain represents the most common cause of disability, and it is the third most common cause of disability in persons aged older than 45 years. By decreasing the body fat, specifically the abdominal or visceral body fat, you place less strain on your back muscles, ligaments, and vertebrae. Primary treatments for low back pain are weight reduction, hamstring stretches, and back and abdominal strengthening exercises. In many cases regular core strengthening exercises can reduce or eliminate back pain completely. Many orthopedic spine surgeons are reluctant to operate on individuals unless they undergo a period of core body strengthening. If one does require back surgery there is evidence that patients with increased core body strength have superior surgical outcomes.

- ***Reduce the Risk of Premature Death:*** Maintaining excellent physical health through exercise decreases effects of hormones on the heart. Hormones can affect the heart by creating serious arrhythmias. Exercise performed regularly with enhancement of aerobic capacity increases heart rate variability, which in turn decreases the risk for sudden death from heart arrhythmias.

- ***Reduce the Risk of Developing and/or Dying from Heart Disease:*** Studies have shown repeatedly that lack of exercise is a risk factor in arterial disease and that moderate to high levels of physical activity reduce coronary heart disease and stroke.

- ***Reduce Depression and Anxiety:*** Regular physical activity and physical fitness are positively associated with mental health and well-being. Persons who are regularly active report less anxiety and depression and lower levels of stress than do sedentary persons. Exercise programs may be useful as an adjunctive therapy for treating mild-to-moderate depression.

- ***Reduce Arthritic Pain***: Both osteoarthritis and rheumatoid arthritis may respond to exercise programs. A sensible training program often significantly reduces the pain associated with these ailments.

Summary: The foregoing are some of the physiologic benefits of performing regular exercise. In addition, exercise has been shown to aid in decreasing the risk of developing and/or reducing the effects of: Alzheimer's disease, peripheral vascular disease, chronic sinusitis, cholelithiasis (gallstones), fibromyalgia, prostate cancer, rheumatoid arthritis, premenstrual syndrome, peripheral neuropathy, urinary tract infections, stroke, peptic ulcer disease, Parkinson's disease, irritable bowel syndrome, menopause, memory loss, macular degeneration, hepatitis, hypothyroidism, gastroesophageal reflux disease, congestive heart failure, and attention deficient disorder. Exercise has been shown to enhance the body physically, create mental and physiologic relaxation, improve mood, and develop mind-body coordination. Consequently, combining strength and endurance training is an effective means for increasing our physical capacity, improving our athletic performance, reducing our injury risk, enhancing our personal appearance, and improving our self-confidence. Essentially, everyone can benefit from a sensible program of exercise.

Additional Further Reading:

1. *Control High Blood Pressure Without Drugs : A Complete Hypertension Handbook* by Robert Rowan, Constance Schrader, 368 pages, Publisher: Fireside; Rev&Updtd ed (May 15, 2001), ISBN: 0684873281

2. *Do You Really Need Back Surgery? : A Surgeon's Guide to Neck and Back Pain and How to Choose Your Treatment* by Aaron G. Filler, 352 pages, Publisher: Oxford University Press (July 15, 2004), ISBN: 0195158350

3. *Handbook of Obesity: Etiology and Pathophysiology* by George Bray, 1072 pages, Publisher: Dekker; 2nd ed (December 9, 2003), ISBN: 0824709691

4. *Harvard Medical School Guide to Lowering Your Cholesterol* by Mason W. Freeman, Christine E. Junge, 272 pages, Publisher: McGraw-Hill; 1st ed (February 10, 2005), ISBN: 0071444815

5. *Hormonal Balance: Understanding Hormones, Weight, and Your Metabolism* by Scott Isaacs, 397 pages, Publisher: Bull Publishing Company; 1st ed (August, 2002), ISBN: 0923521690

6. *Mayo Clinic on Arthritis* by Mayo Clinic, Gene G. Hunder, 198 pages, Publisher: Kensington Publishing Corporation; 2nd ed (October, 2002), ISBN: 1893005259

7. *Muscle Physiology and Cardiac Function* by Lincoln E. Ford, 418 pages, Publisher: Cooper Publishing Group (October 5, 2000), ISBN: 1884125727

8. *Obesity: Etiology, Assessment, Treatment, and Prevention* by Ross E., Ph.D. Andersen, 301 pages, Publisher: Human Kinetics Publishers (June, 2003), ISBN: 0736003282

9. *Preventing and Reversing Osteoporosis : What You Can Do About Bone Loss--A Leading Expert's Natural Approach to Increasing Bone Mass* by Alan Gaby, 320 pages, Publisher: Prima Lifestyles; Reissue ed (April 19, 1995), ISBN: 0761500227

10. *Skeletal Muscle in Health and Disease : A Textbook of Muscle Physiology* by David Jones, Dorothy A. Jones, J. M. Round, 224 pages, Publisher: Manchester University Press (September 15, 1990), ISBN: 0719031648

11. *Skeletal Muscle Metabolism in Exercise and Diabetes* by Erik A. Richter, Bente Kiens, Henrik Galbo, Bengt Saltin, 344 pages, Publisher: Springer; 1st ed (August 31, 1998), ISBN: 0306459205

12. *The Osteoporosis Cure : Reverse the Crippling Effects With New Treatments* by Harris McIlwain, Debra Fulghum Bruce, 208 pages, Publisher: Avon (May 1, 1998), ISBN: 0380793369

CHAPTER 2: How Do I Begin?
(The building blocks of success)

Don't waste life in doubts and fears; spend yourself on the work before you, well assured that the right performance of this hour's duties will be the best preparation for the hours or ages that follow it.
-Ralph Waldo Emerson

The purpose of this chapter is to prepare you to undertake the MAX the MIN Workout. We will talk about goal setting, resources you will need, what to expect from the workout, and when to do it.

Set Goals: When undergoing a major workout program, you should first define your goals. You must be honest and ask yourself, "What is my underlying motivation?" Some people have goals of better fitness, some want healthier lifestyles, some want lean-sculpted figures, while still others are looking for improved performance in their particular sports. Make your goals realistic; you might want to write them down and then set a specific date to begin. You can share your goals with someone, whether a spouse, training partner, etc; who might help you attain it through encouragement.

The road to achieving your goals is not as long as you might imagine. All it takes is knowledge, combined with a little ambition.

The bottom line is to set a goal, commit to it, then do it.

My philosophy of life is that if we make up our minds what we are going to make of our lives, then work hard toward that goal, we never lose - somehow we win out.
-Ronald Reagan

What equipment do you need: You will need access to a pullup bar and a dip bar. These can be found at most gyms, sporting goods stores, or on the internet. A pullup bar can be purchased relatively cheap and placed in a doorframe, a substitute for a dip bar can be made with two chairs in parallel. The best piece of equipment is a combination pullup/dip bar apparatus. Figures 1-4 below illustrate some common pullup and dip equipment.

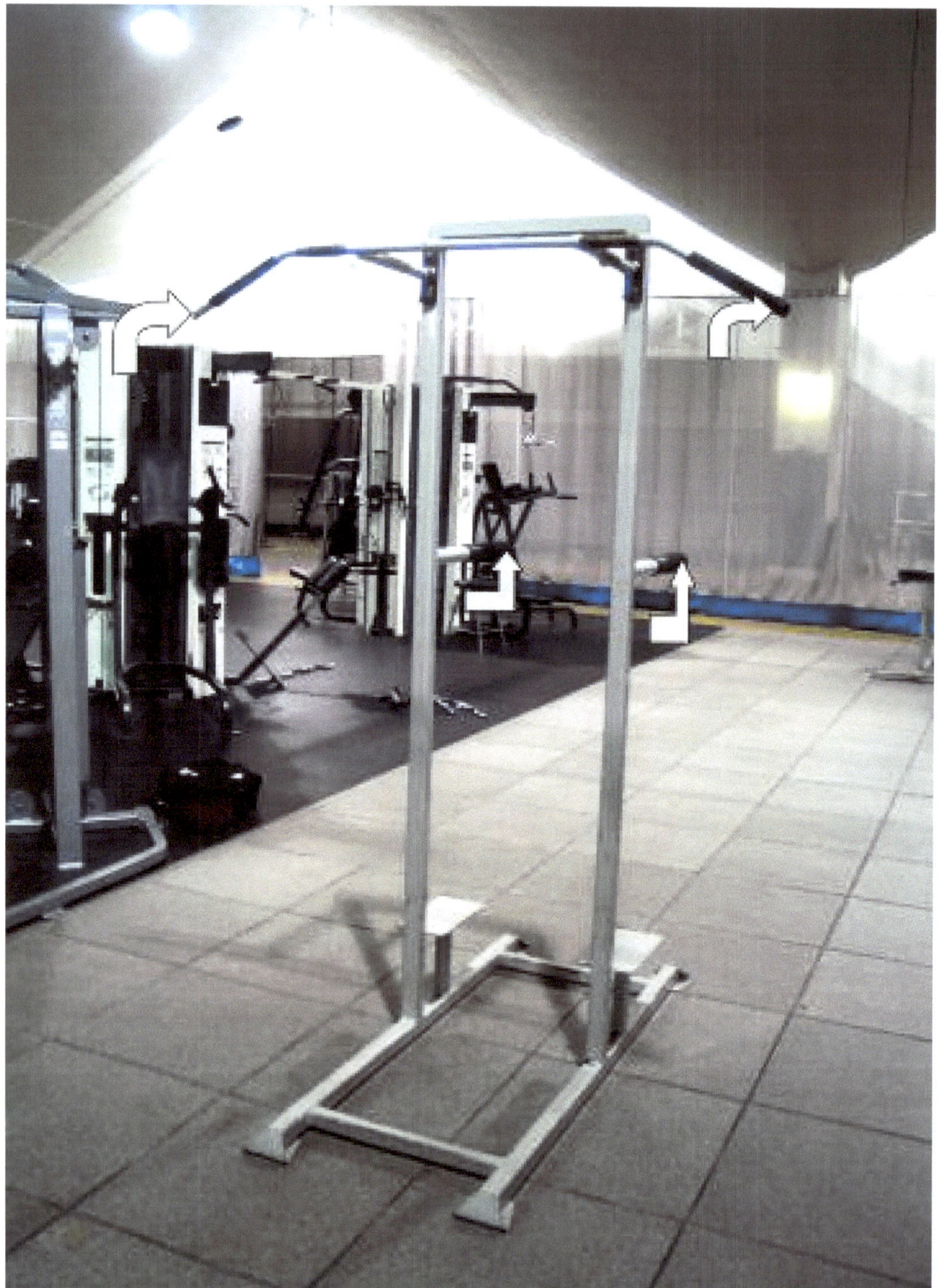

Figure1. A combination pull/dip bar apparatus. Upper arrows point to pullup apparatus. Lower arrows point to dip bars. .

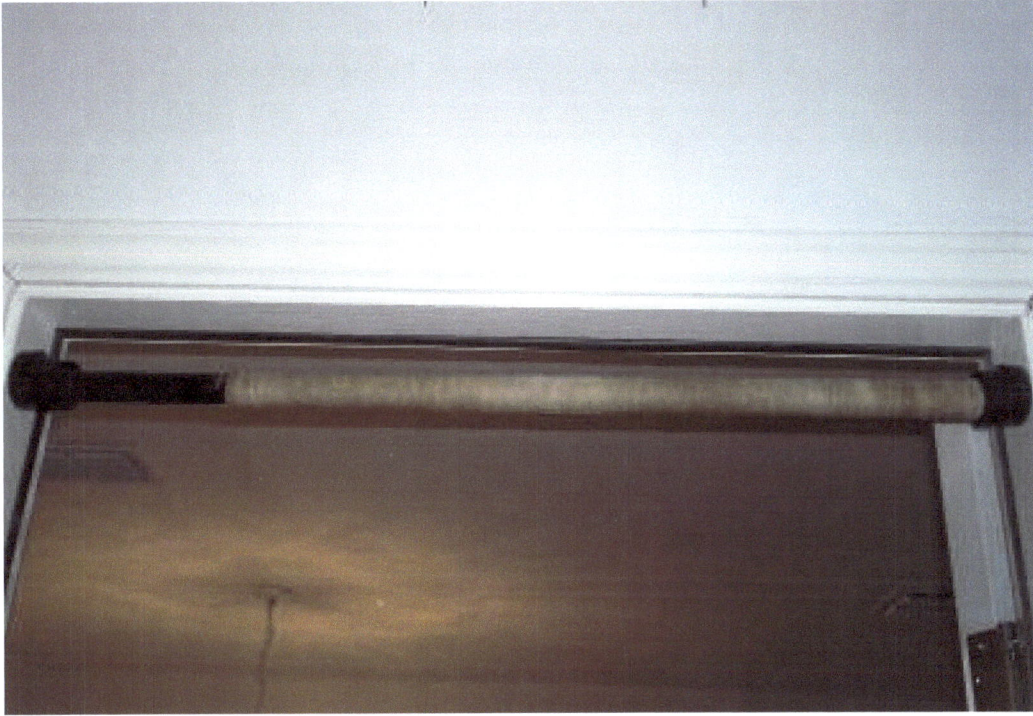

Figure 2. A doorway pullup bar.

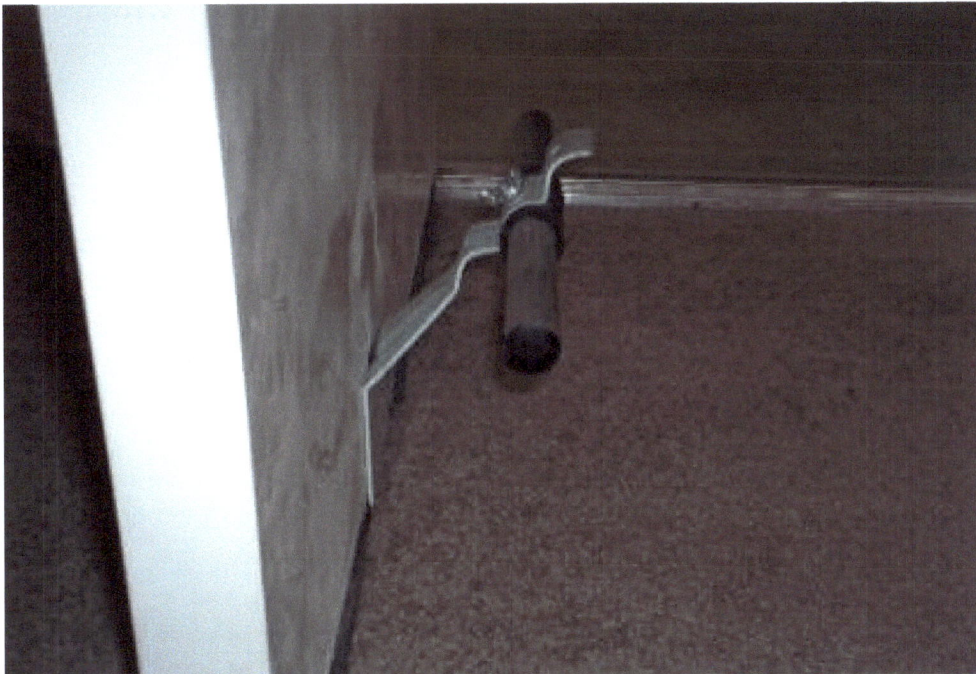

Figure 3. A door situp bar

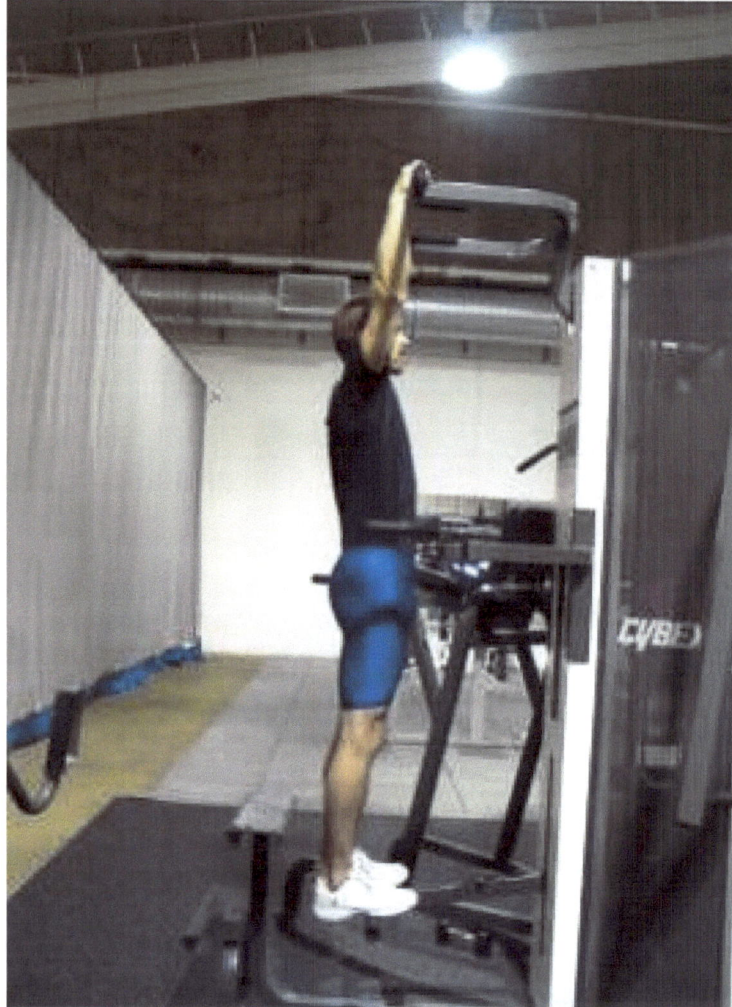

Figure 4. An assisted pullup machine. In this particular assisted pullup/dip combination apparatus, the feet are supported by a bar. The weight can be varied on the support bar to provide a range of difficulties.
..

What to wear: Essentially, dress for comfort. It is best, however, to wear a shirt that will allow you to sweat freely (i.e., a tank top or t-shirt is a good choice you may consider a synthetic fabric which will wick the sweat away from you), comfortable gym shorts and athletic shoes.

How often to workout: A hard and fast recommendation is to work out with these routines **three times a week**. This is in line with research that determined the optimal training frequency of people without heart disease at 3-4 times per week. Additional cardiorespiratory benefits of five or more training sessions per week are minimal while the incidence of injury increases greatly. Although improvements in cardio-respiratory fitness can be seen in people who exercise one to two times per week, such regimens evoke little or no change in fat stores or body weight reduction. The workouts should not be done three days in a row. One option could be to do the workout two days in a row then take 1 to 2 days between before completing the third workout. For example, if you have weekends free for working out, one routine could be completed on Saturday, and then another on Sunday followed by 2-3 days resting or cross training before completing the third routine on Wednesday. Alternatively, you could do a Monday/Wednesday/Friday schedule. Do not be alarmed if you miss a session.

Remember, your workout is your chance to renew, refresh and rejuvenate yourself. Your workout time is the reset button to face life's challenges. The MAX the MIN workout usually only requires a small fraction of your time each week, giving little reason for not completing all three workouts every week.

Confidence: Because the time you spend doing the MAX the MIN workout routines will result in an improvement in your appearance, health, and mental state, it will also result in a significant increase in your self confidence. Most aspects of your personal and professional life will be affected. Others will recognize your new appearance and newfound confidence. In today's society such first impressions mean a lot. A fit physique and confidence commands greater respect. People look to others who are fit, lean, and self-assured. This increase in confidences and energy will also increase the feeling that you can handle the obstacles that life presents.

When to do the routine: For many professions it is possible to set aside a particular time of day to workout, but the time of day is up to you. By making your workout times the same everyday it becomes habit. The nice aspect of the MAX the MIN workout is that it can fit into your schedule whenever you have some down time. It is imperative that you do not skip workouts in the first 2 weeks because of feeling physically exhausted. Just like a savings account you must first invest before you can start making withdrawals. You can come back the next day and do the workout. This is one advantage of a three times a week program. If you decided to workout on back-to-back days (e.g. Saturday/Sunday) it is imperative that you do not skip out on parts of the planned program due to feeling tired or sore. You should push yourself through the soreness and tiredness to discover your limits.

This workout will improve your state of mind. A workout in the middle of your working day will enhance your mental acuity and productivity. Some find that the MAX the MIN workout works best in place of lunch since this may be the only time they have to themselves. Indeed, assuming that you eat a healthy breakfast, exercising over the lunch hour will leave you more alert to tackle the afternoon than eating a heavy meal with no exercise. Make sure you save a little time to grab a quick bite to eat after your workout. In the hours following your workout, your appetite will increase and at that time you might want to have a small healthy snack prior to dinner (e.g. yogurt, fruit, and vegetables). Make sure you bring healthy snacks to work, so you don't find yourself raiding the vending machine.

If you workout in the evenings and want to get a good night's sleep, do your workout about two to three hours prior to your desired bedtime. Physical activity will increase your body temperature and make you more alert. As your body temperature lowers following exercise you will find it easier to fall asleep.

What to do on days between workouts: Whatever you like! If you are already doing other sports or workout programs, you can continue to lift weights, run, swim, bicycle, or play any sport. Whether you choose to participate in other activities or take a rest day is your choice.

Many people enjoy running and/or bicycling which helps to strengthen the legs and heart. The distance depends upon what you want to achieve. Some prefer long distances at a slower pace. This will improve endurance and is good cardiovascular training. Like plastic, your body will mold to its usage. So mix it up a little bit. Try some power work in the middle of your long run or bike. Your sprints could be as short as 50 meters and as long as 800 meters. Do not begin sprinting at 100% effort. In fact, it is better to start slow with your first sprint, then increase to 50% effort, then to 75% effort and finish at 90-95% effort. This will reduce the chance of injury. Your next two or three sprints should start off faster. Sprinting will build the muscles in your upper legs. Mixing up your speed during your bike rides or runs will make your body adapt to change, just like it has to in life.

Other people enjoy racket sports including squash, tennis, racquetball, handball, among others. This is a great idea and one where your body constantly has to react. Not only do you develop your cardiovascular system, but your eye-hand coordination also improves.

Rest: Proper rest is essential. As most athletes know, over-training will make you less competitive than under-training. The body builds itself during these periods of rest. Depriving yourself of this will result in continued break down of your body. Days off can be just as important as your most intense training days. Every fourth week and immediately after a test week you should decrease your intensity to 60-70% of your standard workout based on your new set of maximums. This initially might sound counterproductive, but you are engaging in an intense workout program that can lead to over-training. An easy week after three weeks of consistent training will avoid over-training.

Take a day off to refuel. Erase the thought: "I'm lazy if I take a day off." Taking a rest day is being smart, not lazy. Rest days are essential to reduce the risk of injury and provide muscles with time to refuel. Performance improves more with quality exercise not quantity of exercise.

Training Progression: Every training program needs a protocol for progressing in the workout. While it is important to periodically increase the exercise intensity, it is equally important to do so gradually. A safe and productive progression is known as the 10% rule. That is, you never step up the MAX the MIN program more than 10% per week.

For example, if you complete 10 repetitions of an exercise in good form, you should increase the number of repetitions by 10 percent or less for the following week. This means you should strive for 11 repetitions of each exercise. The same holds true for your time intervals. If you complete the exercises within the desired time with time to spare (e.g. 1 minute interval and are getting more than 20 seconds rest you should decrease your time interval by no more than 10% (e.g. 54 seconds). Do not decrease time interval and increase repetitions in the same week unless both added together equal a program that is not more than 10% more difficult.

The 10 % rule provides small but frequent training increments to progressively stress the muscular system. Under no circumstances should repetitions be increased or time interval decreased by more than 10% over a one-week period. Remember it is better to do 10% less with quality as opposed to 10% more.

Training Range: Full range muscle strength is best developed through full range exercise movements. In other words, the training effect is greatest within the exercised portion of the joint movement range. Full range strength reduces injury risk and increases performance potential. Try to perform each repetition through a full range of movement, but never to a position of discomfort. The MAX the MIN workout emphasizes the continuous use of large-muscle groups designing exercises that are rhythmic and aerobic in nature. Research has shown that these types of activities are the most effective and lend themselves to individualized specific exercises prescriptions.[43]

Just prior to working out: Stretch lightly prior to beginning any workout. It is important that you begin slowly and progress to harder exercises. The first few pullups, dips, pushups, situps, etc. often seem to be difficult. You may even wish to do a few warm up sets followed by stretching before you begin the actual workout for that day. The warm up sets will increase blood flow to your musculature and allow stretching to be more effective. As your body warms up, these will seem to get easier.

Breathing: Focus on your breathing during your workout. Make your breathing match your exercise. For example, if you are doing pushups breathe in on the downward phase and breathe out on the upward phase. For situps, breathe in as you let yourself down and breathe out as you sit back up.

During your workout: It is essential to continually keep your muscles loose while engaged in your workout. This may consist of "shaking" out your arms after a set or swinging them in a few circles after your set. This reduces the amount of muscle spasm and increases the blood flow to the muscles. As you near the end of your workout it will become more challenging. This is when you have to commit to finishing.

Doing your workout with others: A workout program done with others strengthens your commitment to both beginning and finishing. Having partners provides an atmosphere for accomplishment, improvement and accountability. You are responsible to your partner and they are responsible to you. Be supportive and encouraging to one another while making sure that you are completing the exercises in the specified time interval. Positive reinforcement rather than negative comments almost always results in a better performance.

However, do not let conversation interfere with the workout or completion in a specified time period. At times you may be tempted to take a break and talk about the days' events. Resist this urge if it interferes with your workout and decreases your heart rate below your zone. This is your time to get the most out of a workout. Just having someone doing the exercises with you will be a significant amount of support in itself.

What to expect: Over time, you may develop calluses on your hands from some of the exercises. If this bothers you, wear workout gloves. It will take a minimum of two weeks for your body to adapt to your new strenuous workout program. As the weeks go by, your body will adapt and you will be able to complete more repetitions in a shorter period of time. After about two weeks of strict adherence to the guidelines set forth, you will experience improvement in your strength and ability to accomplish given exercises.

It will take approximately six weeks to see results in your body shape and composition. Your muscles respond to the stress you place on them by becoming stronger, yet the changes must happen microscopically before you can see them. Larger changes take more time. It is important to stay vigilant and focused during the first several weeks. Historically, the first few weeks are the time period when it is easiest to give-up. At around six weeks you will notice changes in your body. Your body is reorganizing itself in response to the requirements you have placed on it. You may want to take a photo of yourself prior to your workout program and then after six weeks of working out consistently. The before and after photos will show your progress and reinforce your dedication. As the workout becomes easier, it is important to increase the number of repetitions or decrease the time interval for finishing a given workout to keep the intensity high.

Vary Your Routine: Doing the same routine can often become boring or tedious. Introduce variety and change to your workout on a weekly or monthly basis. Personalize your workout with the exercises you enjoy most.

Perform one single set at your maximum ability each month. That is, perform one set of each exercise at your maximum ability. Try to push yourself beyond that which you previously accomplished. The purpose of testing yourself is to check your progress, document your improvement, and ensure you are training in the proper zones and ability.

The first time you test yourself you might see a slight decrease in the number of maximum repetitions that you can complete. Do not despair, you are supposed to be fatigued and your muscles are tired. By your second round of testing the increases you have been looking for will be there. In fact, for the first several months of testing you may see dramatic increases in the maximum number of repetitions you can perform. This is because the high-repetition, stamina and muscle building exercises that the MAXimize the MINimum workout emphasizes are making your muscles more efficient than they have been before. Over time, you will begin to plateau and the dramatic increases will taper. During this time it is critical to maintain your vigilance and make sure you are increasing the workouts to keep the intensity at a high level while not increasing your workout more than 10% per week.

Time Yourself: It is very important to time yourself so that you complete your workout within a set time period. The amount of time you spend on a routine will depend upon your everyday demands and time you have available. The MAX the MIN workout is designed to be accomplished in 30 to 60 minutes. However, some elite athletes may spend up to 2 hours on it. Set aside time to dress, workout, shower, and redress. Interval timing is the key to success in this program. You should wear a watch to monitor your time. Some individuals set the countdown timer function on their stopwatches to gauge their progress through the routine. By maintaining an interval you keep your heart rate elevated throughout the entire workout. Research has shown little additional cardiovascular benefit beyond 30-minute sessions, excluding warm-up and cool-down.

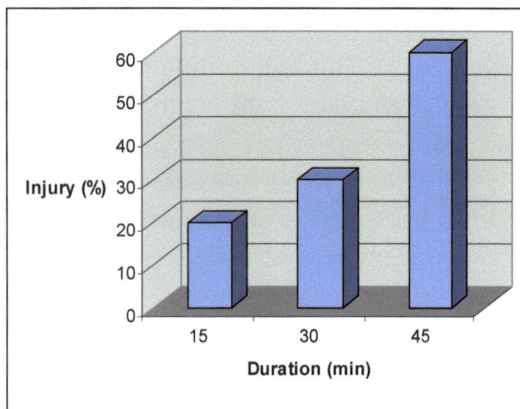

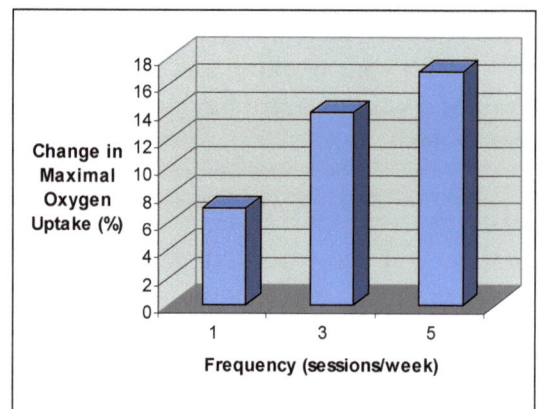

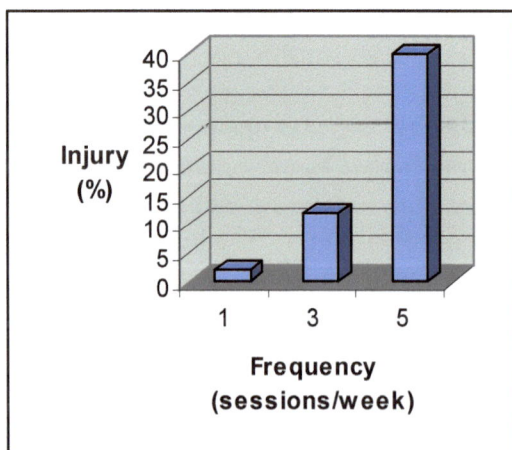

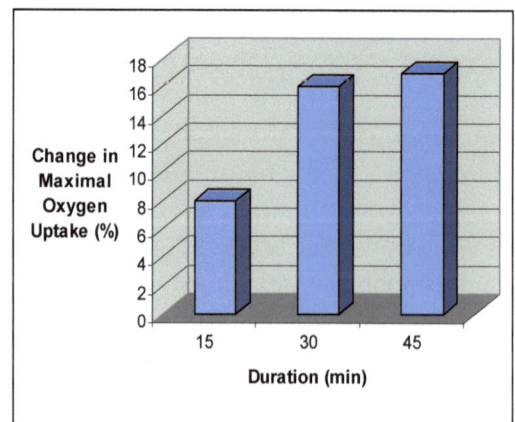

Relationship between exercise frequency and duration, improvement in maximal oxygen consumption and the incidence of orthopaedic injury. Above an exercise duration of 3 sessions a week, additional improvement in maximal oxygen consumption is small and injury rate increases disproportionately. (Data from Pollock ML, Gettman LR, Milesis CA et al: Effects of frequency and duration of training on attrition and incidence of injury. Med Sci Sports 9:31-36, 1977.)

Pyramiding: Pyramiding is another way to maximize your effort. Essentially, this involves starting an exercise easily and getting progressively harder until a limit is reached. You can then gradually decrease the effort to easier sets.

For example, with sets of pushups, you can start with two and progress to four, then six, etc. until a maximum predetermined amount is reached, and then gradually decrease the number of pushups per set by two (e.g. 2,4,6,8,10, 8,6,4,2. By pyramiding your sets you essentially build into your workout a warm-up and cool-down into the set.

Ladders: A ladder is the same principle as a pyramid, but you do not do the back side of the pyramid. You begin with easier sets and progress to more difficult sets. Or you may choose to do a reverse ladder and progress from difficult sets to easier sets.

An example of a ladder might be pushups when you start with 2 and progress is increments of 2 until you reach 20.

Injury: You may feel fatigued and sore when first starting a workout program. After about one week the fatigue will begin to lessen. All significant soreness should have dissipated by week two. If you feel that you have suffered a strain, either from something you have done, or while completing the routine, a generally accepted rule of thumb is the "Rule of seven:" following a strain or sprain, take seven days of rest, ice, elevation and an anti-inflammatory medication (e.g. ibuprofen), followed by seven days of lighter intensity workout before starting back into the regular routine. If an injury hurts for greater than this amount of time, you should see a physician.

While anti-inflammatory agents are available over-the-counter, these medications can be associated with serious side effects, especially if used in large quantities for prolonged periods of time. Consult the manufacturer's guidelines and talk to your physician before beginning any medication.

Training Exercises: Perhaps the most important aspect of a well-designed strength-training program is to address all of the major muscle groups. A comprehensive training approach produces overall strength development and reduces the risk of muscle imbalance injuries. The target muscle groups of many exercises are listed in the following table.

Exercise	Major Muscle Groups
Predominately Upper Body Exercises	
Pushup	Pectoralis Major, Triceps, Deltoids, Paraspinal
Pullup	Latissimus Dorsi, Deltoids, Triceps, Paraspinal
Chin up	Latissimus Dorsi, Deltoids, Biceps, Paraspinal
Dip	Pectoralis Major, Deltoids, Triceps
Predominately Lower Body Exercises	
Lunges	Quadriceps, Hamstrings, Gluteals

Stiff Leg Deadlift	Hamstrings
Squat Jumps	Quadriceps, Gluteals
Box Jumps	Quadriceps, Gastrocnemious, Gluteals
Ski Jumpers	Quadriceps, Gastrocnemious, Gluteals
Air Squats	Quadriceps, Gluteals
Iron Mike's	Quadriceps, Gluteals

Core Exercises/Total Body

Sit up	Rectus Abdominis
V up	Rectus Abdominis
Jumping Jacks	Gastrocnemious/Quadriceps/Deltoids
Superman's	Paraspinal/Gluteals
Leg Raises	Rectus Abdominis
Hanging Leg Raises	Rectus Abdominis, External Oblique
Flutter Kicks	Rectus Abdominis/Hip Flexors
Hello Dolly's	Rectus Abdominis/Hip Flexors
Windshield Wipers	Rectus Abdominis/External Oblique
Halo Jumpers	Paraspinal/Gluteals
Hanging Leg Raises	Rectus Abdominis
Air Up	Paraspinal
Mad Hubbert's	Rectus Abdominis/Hip Flexors

Shoulders

Chest

Biceps

Abdominals

Forearms

Quadriceps

Tibialis
Anterior

Trapezius

Triceps

Lats

Lower Back

Glutes

Hamstrings

Calves

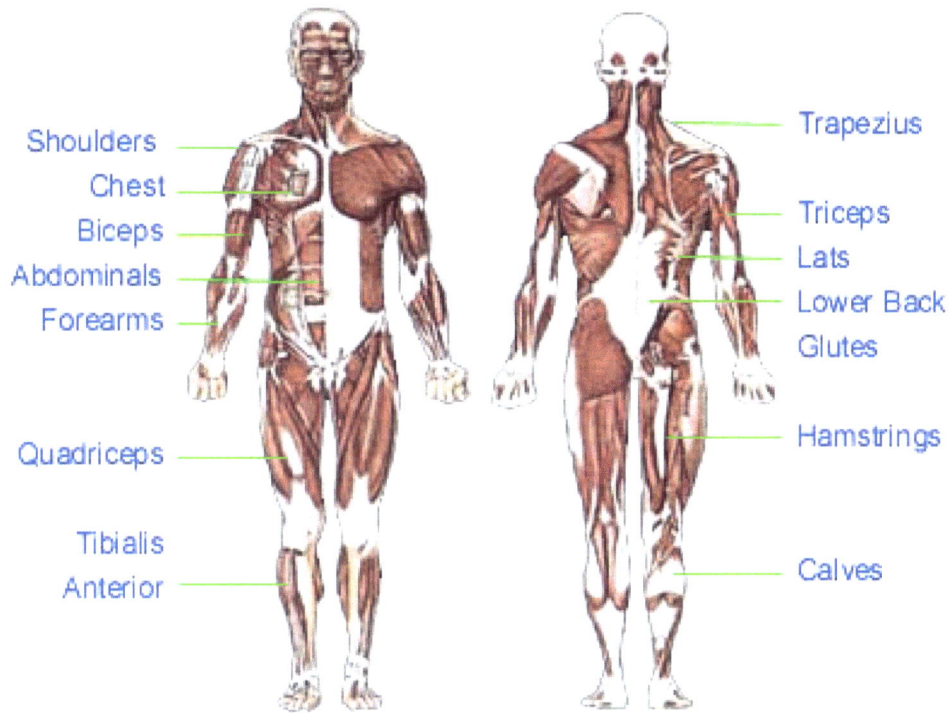

Additional Further Reading:

1. *Goal Setting 101 : How to Set and Achieve a Goal!*
   by Gary Ryan Blair, 58 pages, Publisher: Blair Pub House (June 8, 2000), ISBN: 1889770647
2. *Motivation and Goal Setting: How to Set and Achieve Goals and Inspire Others*
   by Jim Cairo, 128 pages, Publisher: Career Press; 1st ed (July, 1998), ISBN: 1564143643
3. *The Promise of Sleep: A Pioneer in Sleep Medicine Explores the Vital Connection Between Health, Happiness, and a Good Night's Sleep*
   by William C. Dement, Christopher Vaughan, 512 pages, Publisher: Dell (March 7, 2000), ISBN: 0440509017
4. *The Ultimate Secrets of Total Self-Confidence*
   by Robert Anthony, 240 pages, Publisher: Berkley (November 15, 1986), ISBN: 0425101703

I know the price of success: dedication, hard work and an unremitting devotion to the things you want to see happen.
-Frank Lloyd Wright

PROPER FORM: To learn the proper form for doing the exercises, a picture is worth a thousand words. The following photos will illustrate the correct positions for doing the different exercises recommend in this text.

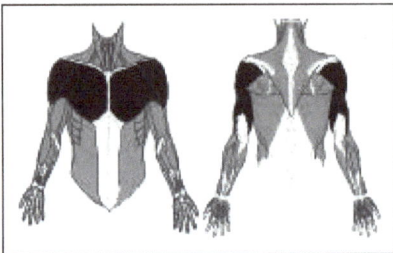

Standard Push Up

Beginning Phase: Lower body towards the floor until chest just touches floor, while keeping back parallel to the floor (Figure below).

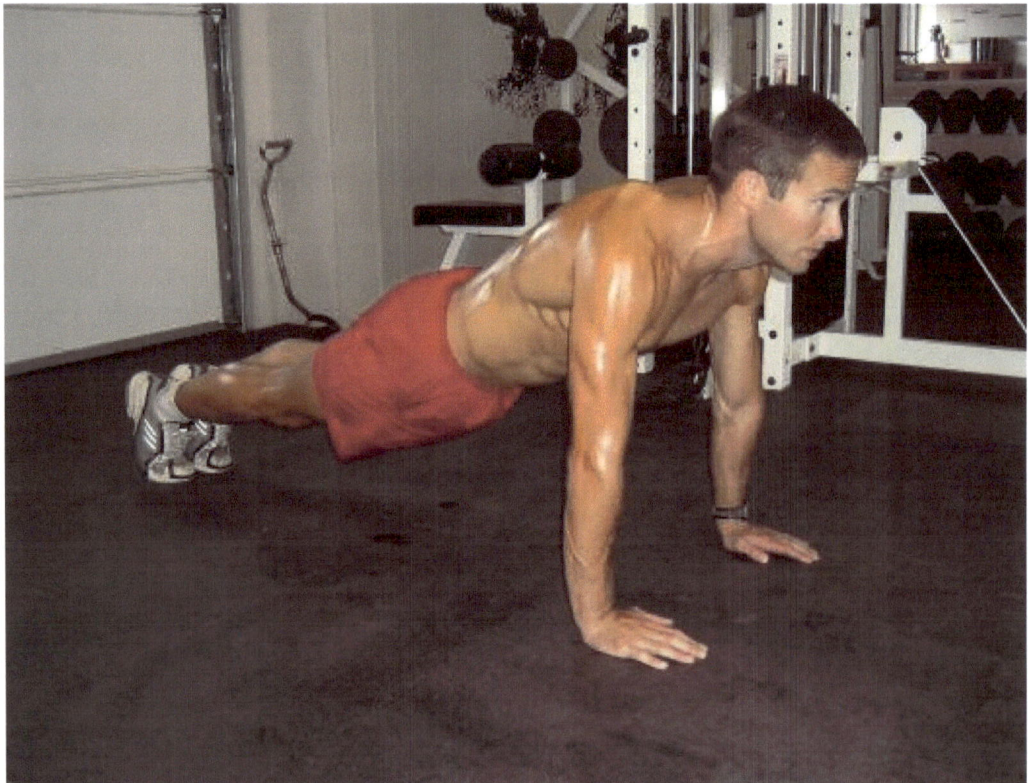

Movement Phase: Lower body towards the floor until your elbows reach a 90-degree angle, while keeping back parallel to the floor (Figure below).

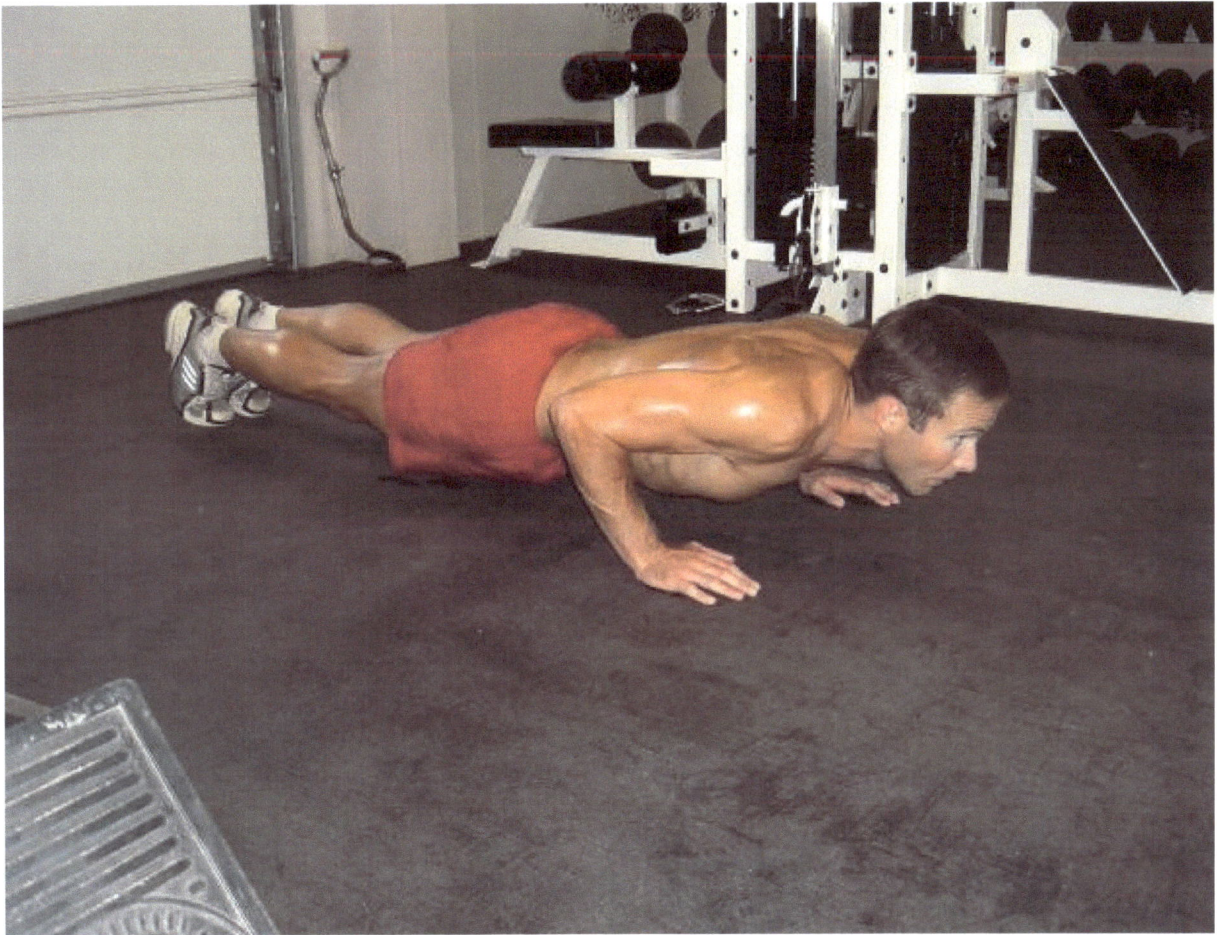

Ending Phase: Push your body back to starting position slowly and with control until your elbows are extended.

❗ TIPS

✓ Keep your head up and focus your eyes on an object in front of you. Do not look at the ground.

✓ Do not bend your knees or let your back sag. Flex your gluteal muscles (butt muscles) and tighten your abs, this will help straighten out your knees and back.

✓ Breathe in as you lower yourself and breathe out as you raise yourself.

✓ Focus on the set as a whole, and not on any single pushup. Avoid pausing at any time. If you must pause, pause in the 'up' position with elbows extended.

✓ Avoid jerky movements. Instead, do the repetitions in a graceful manner.

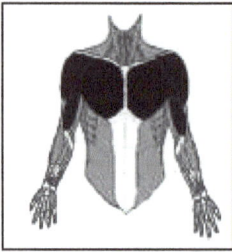

Wide Push Up

Beginning Phase: Start facing the floor with arms extended about 1 hand breath wider than shoulder width on each side, back flat and feet together (Figure below).

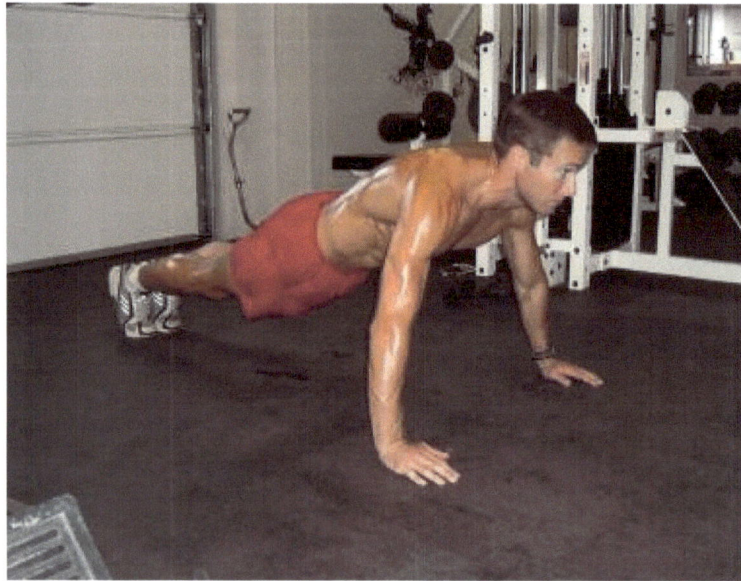

Movement Phase: Lower body towards the floor until your elbows form a 90-degree angle, while keeping back parallel to the floor (Figure below).

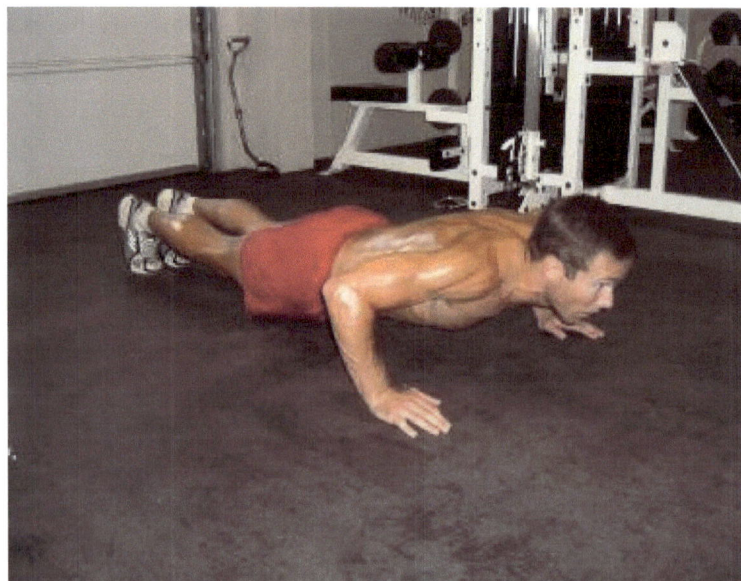

Ending Phase: Push your body back to starting position slowly and with control until your elbows are fully extended.

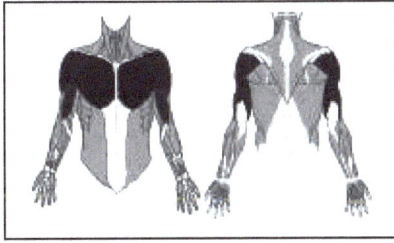

Diamond Push Up

Beginning Phase: Start facedown on the floor with hands forming a 'diamond' position centered directly below your chest, back flat and feet together (Figure below).

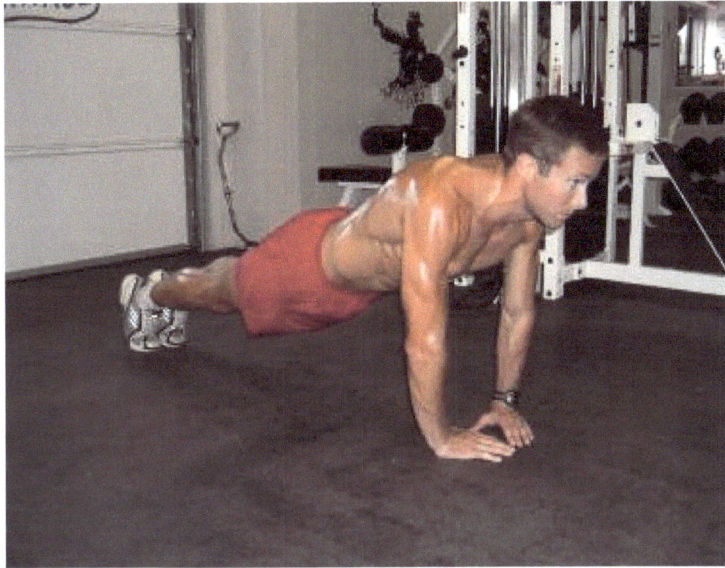

Movement Phase: Lower body towards the floor until your elbows form a 90-degree angle, while keeping back parallel to the floor (Figure below).

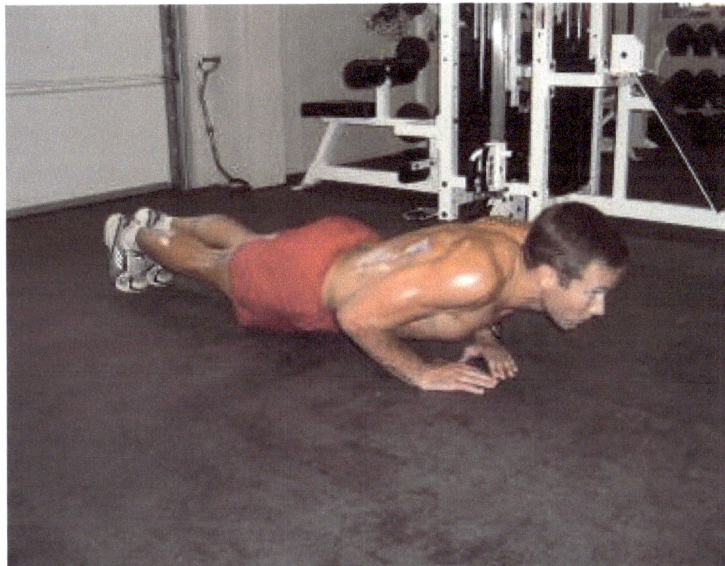

Ending Phase: Push your body back to starting position slowly and with control until your elbows are fully extended.

Beginner's Push Ups

Same as regular push-ups, except knees, rather than toes, are on floor.

Beginning Phase: Start facing the floor with arms extended, shoulder width apart, back flat, feet together, and knees on floor (Figure below).

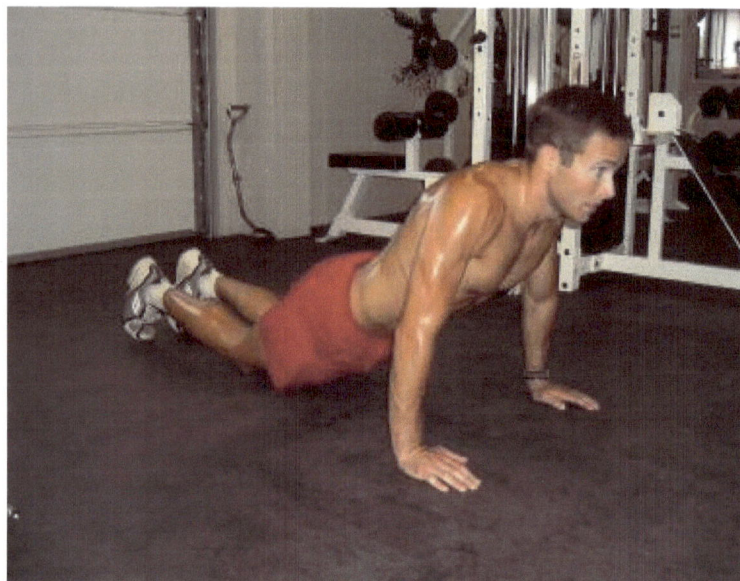

Movement Phase: Lower body towards the floor until your elbows make a 90-degree angle, while keeping back parallel to the floor (Figure below).

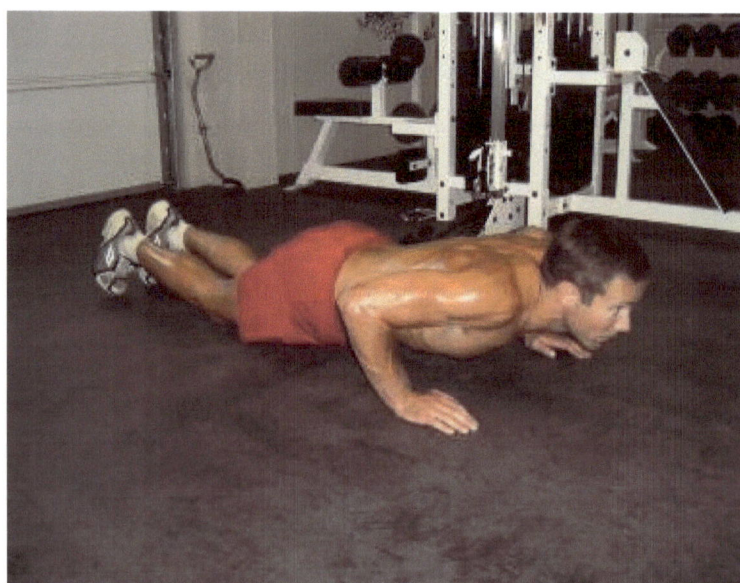

Ending Phase: Push your body back to starting position slowly and with control until your elbows are fully extended.

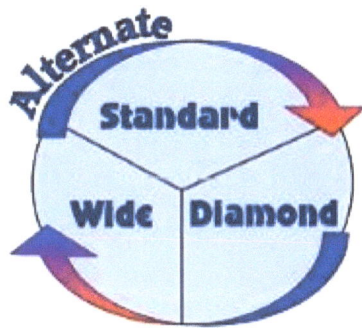

Push up examples sets

Beginner
6x10   45 second time interval

Intermediate
6x25   45 second time interval

Hard
6x50   50 second time interval

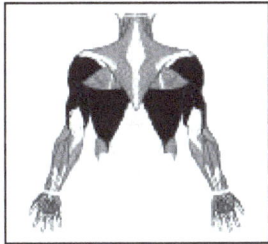

Standard Pull Up

Beginning Phase: Grasp the bar with palms facing away. Your hands should be at about the width of your shoulders apart (Figure below).

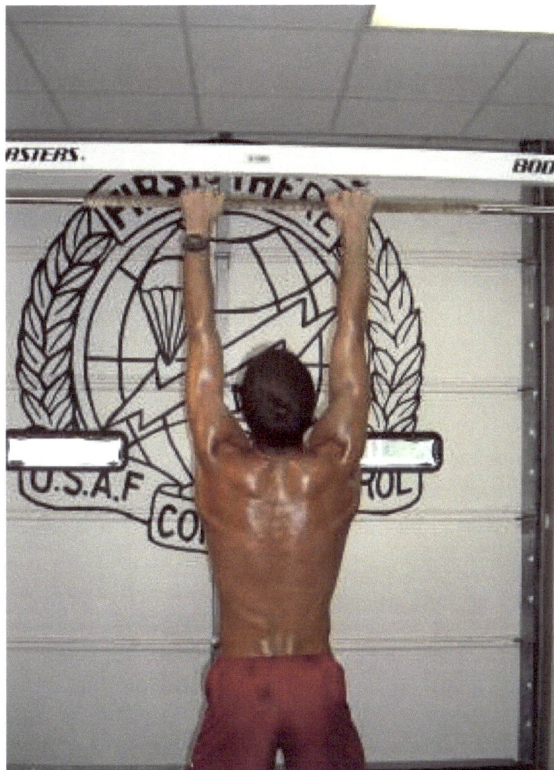

Upward Phase: With torso erect, eyes fixed forward and arms fully extended slowly pull until your chin rises above the bar (Figure below).

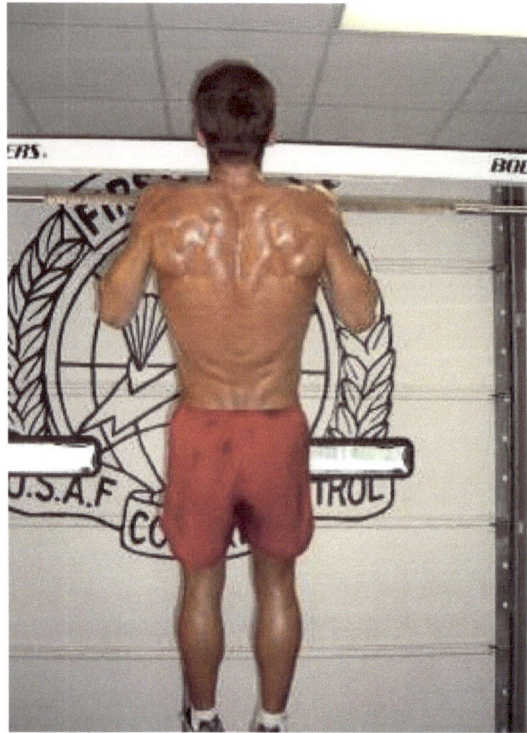

Downward Phase: Control the descent back into the starting position allowing the arms to fully extend.

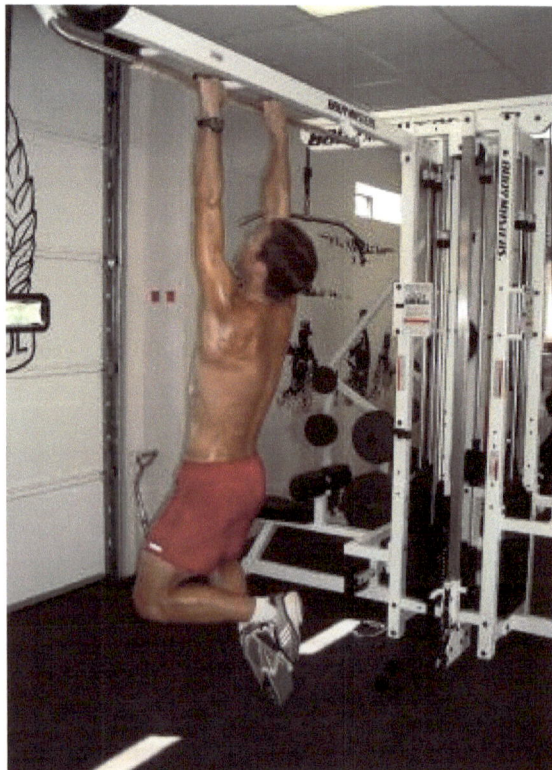

TIPS Always grip the bar with the thumb on top (Figure below).

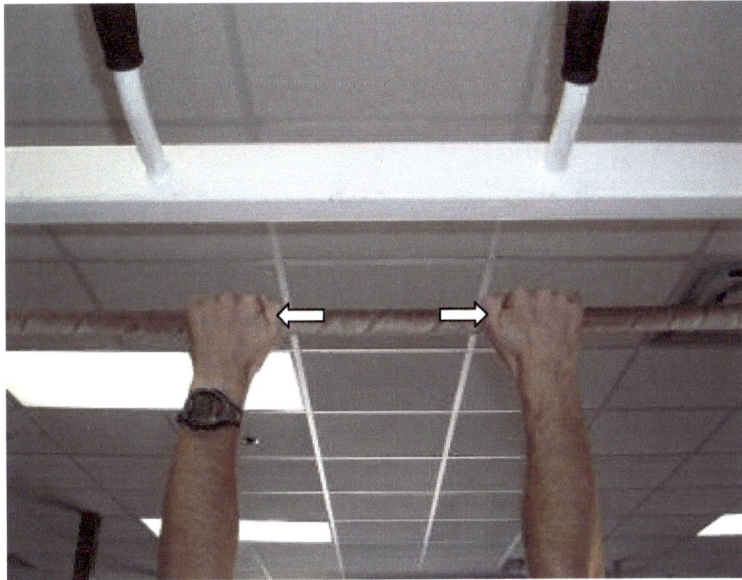

TIPS ✓ Think of sets as a group and do not solely concentrate on each repetition.

✓ Follow your body's natural rhythm during the upward and downward phases.

✓ Focus your eyes on an object in the distance and watch that object to control your head position as you pull your body up.

✓ Breathe in as you pull yourself up, and breathe out as you let yourself down.

✓ Do not pause. Keep in constant motion. If you must pause, pause in the 'down' position with elbows extended.

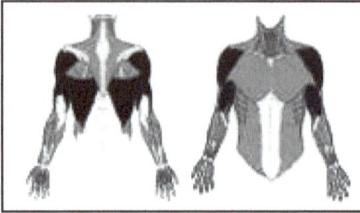

Wide Grip Pull Up

Beginning Phase: Grasp the bar with palms facing away. Your hands should be placed two hand widths wider than the width of your shoulders (Figure below).

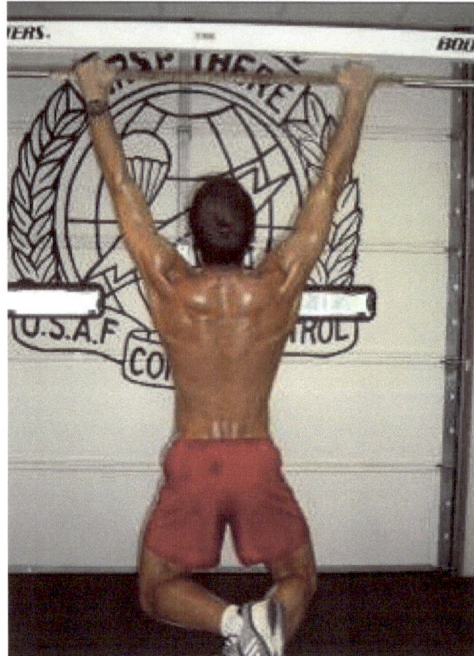

Upward Phase: With torso erect, eyes fixed forward and arms fully extended slowly pull until your chin rises above the bar (Figure below).

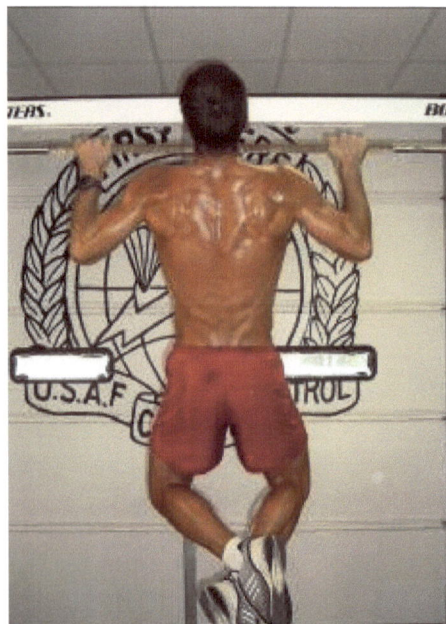

Downward Phase: Control the descent back into the starting position allowing the arms to fully extend.

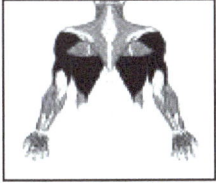

Close Grip Pull Up

Beginning Phase: Grasp the bar with palms facing away. Your hands should be placed together with thumbs touching (Figure below).

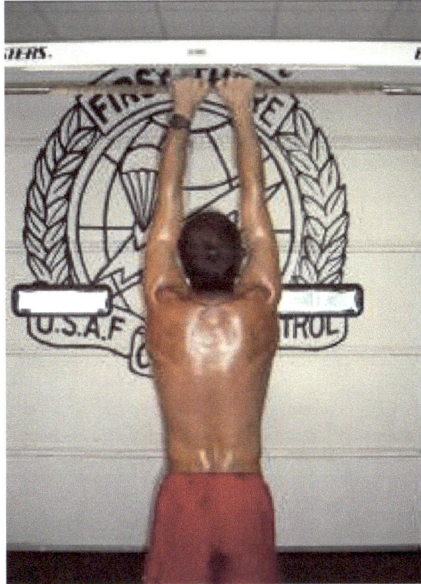

Upward Phase: With torso erect, eyes fixed forward and arms fully extended slowly pull until your chin rises above the bar (Figure below).

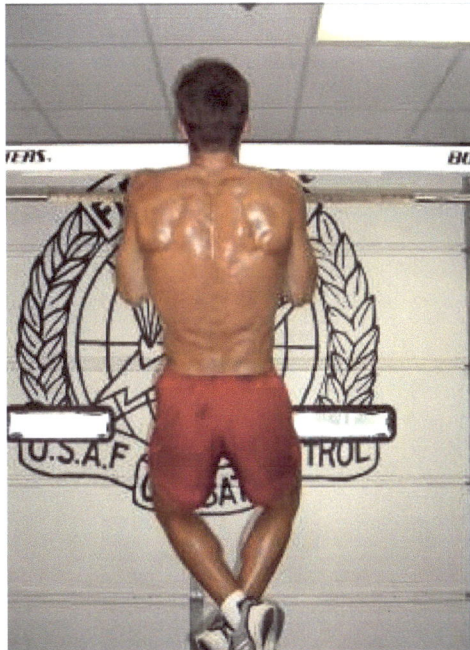

Downward Phase: Control the descent back into the starting position allowing the arms to fully extend.

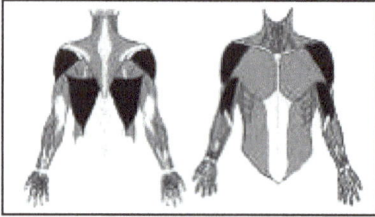

Chin-Up

Beginning Phase: Grasp the bar with palms facing toward you. Your hands should be at about the width of your shoulders apart (Figure below).

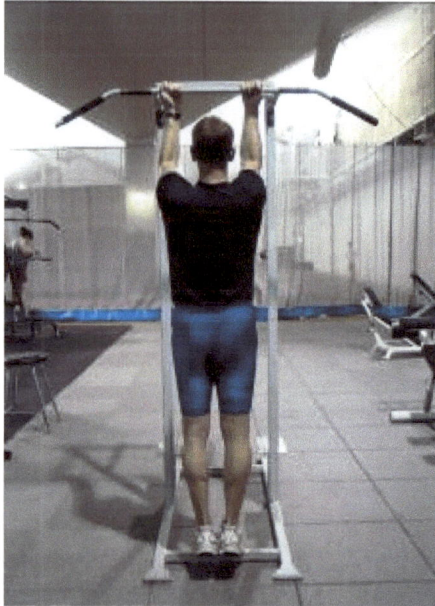

Upward Phase: With torso erect, eyes fixed forward and arms fully extended slowly pull until your chin rises above the bar (Figure below).

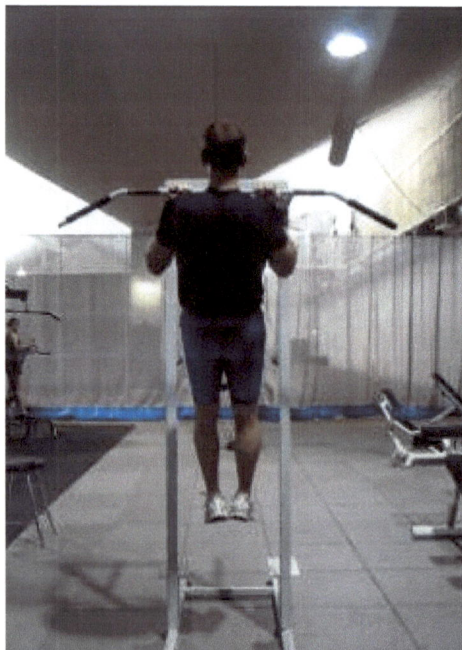

Downward Phase: Control the descent back into the starting position allowing the arms to fully extend.

Combination (i.e., cross-grip) Pull-up/Chin-up

Beginning Phase: Use the handgrip of the pull-up with one hand while gripping the bar with the handgrip of a chin-up with the other (Figure below).

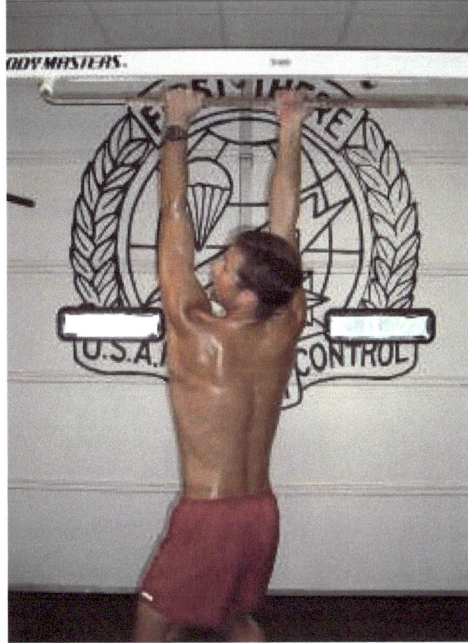

Upward Phase: With torso erect, eyes fixed forward and arms fully extended slowly pull until your chin rises above the bar (Figure below).

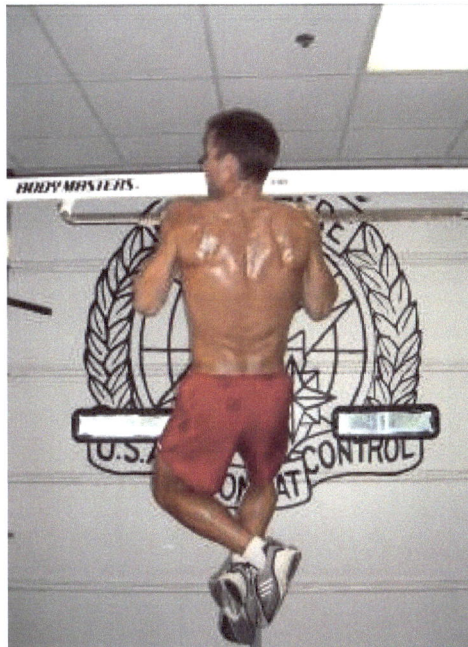

Downward Phase: Control the descent back into the starting position allowing the arms to fully extend.

❗ Alternate grips to work both sides

Assisted Pull-ups/Chin-ups

The grip is the same as the standard pull-up; however, the exercise is accomplished either with a pull-up assist machine or by a partner clasping the legs or torso (Figure below).

It is critical that good communication is established as the person performing the exercise begins to fatigue. If the assisting partner is holding the legs they must be released in time to prevent injury.

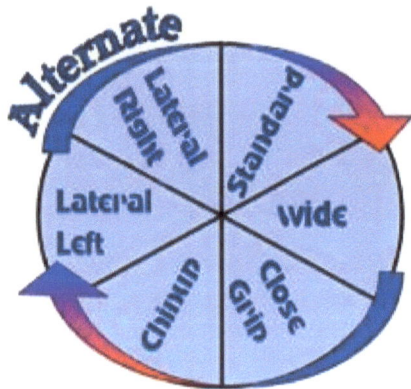

Pull up examples sets

Beginner
6x3   45 second time interval

Intermediate
6x7   45 second time interval

Hard
6x15   60 second time interval

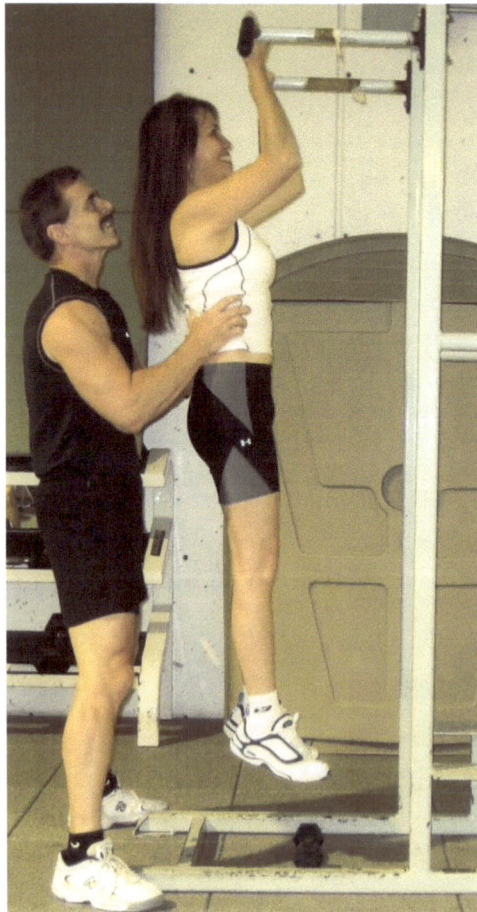

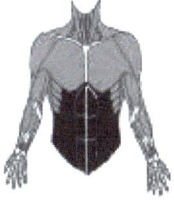

The Oblique Sit Up

Beginning Phase: Lie face up on a soft surface, bend knees and bring feet close to the buttocks. Interlock fingers behind or on top of head (Figure below).

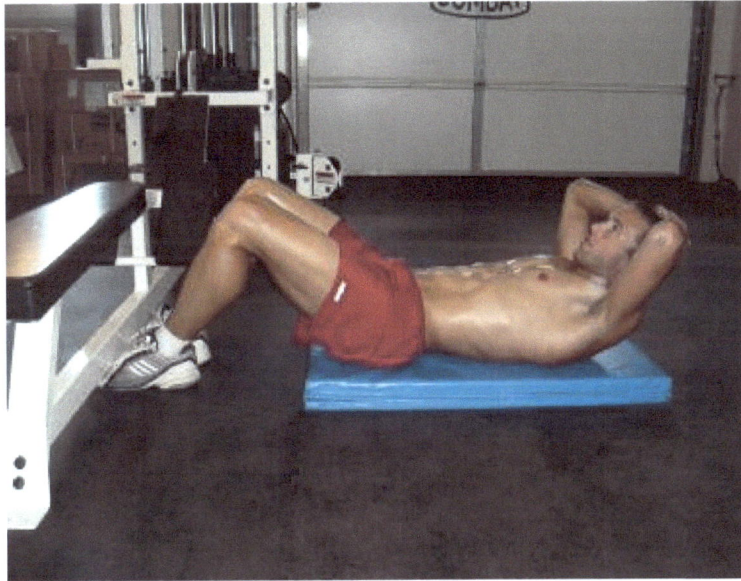

Upward Movement: With abdominal muscles, begin lifting your upper body and twisting while reaching for your opposite knee (Figures below).

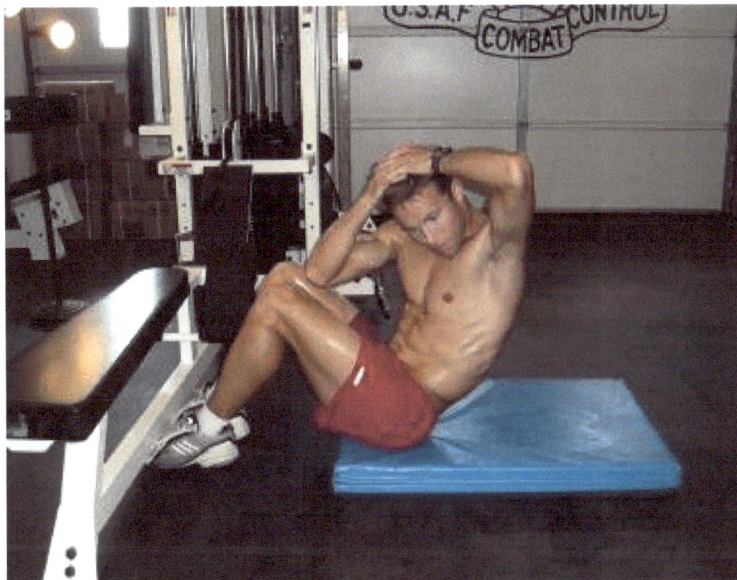

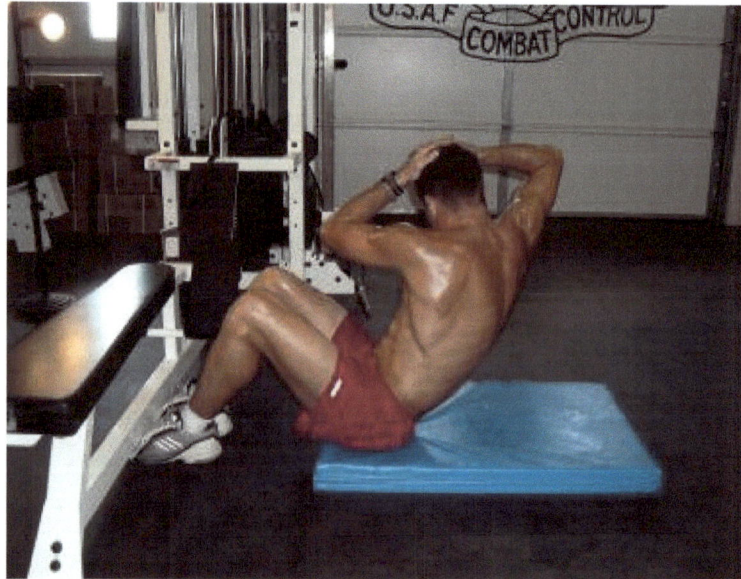

Downward Movement: Lower shoulders and upper body slowly and with control until small of back touches floor.

Standard Sit Up: In the standard sit up, your legs are only slightly bent and you do not reach for the opposite knee.

❗ TIPS

✓ Placing your hands on top of your head as opposed to behind your head so you do not pull with your arms and strain on your neck (Figure below).

✓ Tuck your toes in anywhere you can find. Benches, ledges, and couches all work great.

✓ Watch the angle formed by your knee. Keeping it less than 90-degrees uses more abdominal muscles (rectus abdominis, external oblique), while an angle greater than 90-degrees uses more hip flexor muscles (iliospoas) (Figure below).

✓ Pretend there is an apple between your chin and chest to keep from putting too much stain on your neck.

✓ Having your hands on top of your head increases the difficulty of the sit up because more weight is further displaced from your center of gravity. If sit ups with your hands on your head are too difficult, cross arms across chest as this makes your center of gravity more centralized. However, the idea is to have your hands and arms as far from where you bend at the waist as possible for a more challenging workout.

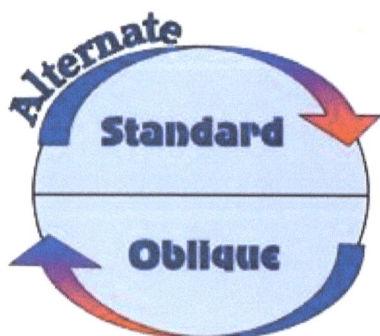

Alternate Standard / Oblique

Sit up examples sets

Beginner
6x15 (x3 for each set) **45 second time interval**

Intermediate
6x25 (x3 for each set) **45 second time interval**

Hard
6x45 (x3 for each set) **60 second time interval**

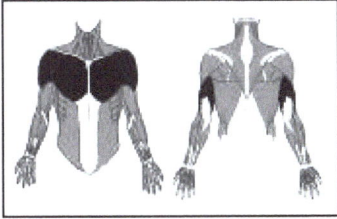

Dip

Beginning Position: Hands gripping bar, upper body erect, eyes fixed forward (Figure below).

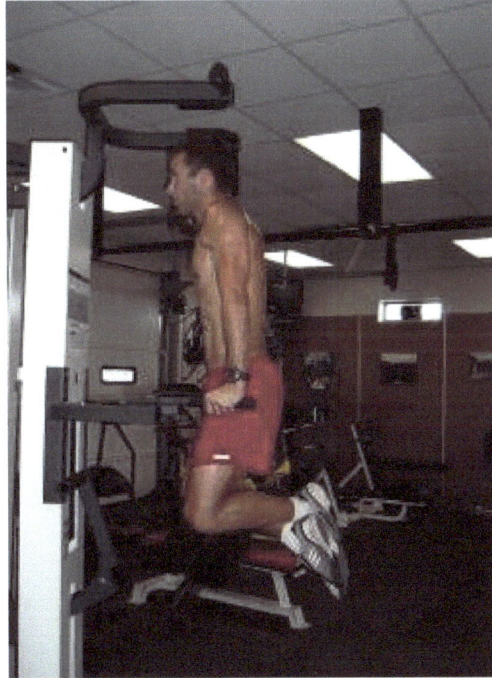

Downward Movement Phase: Bend arms to nearly a 90-degree angle, keep body erect, eyes fixed forward (Figure below).

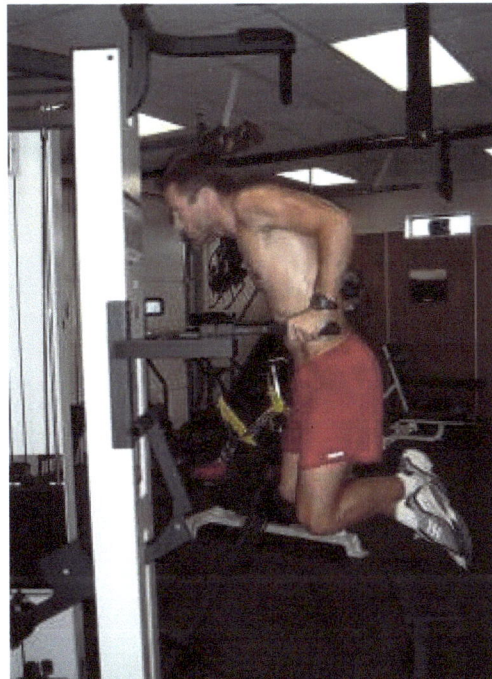

Upward Movement Phase: Fully straighten arms again, keep body erect, head facing forward.

35

✓ Do not go beyond 90 degrees of elbow flexion.

✓ Do not pause. If you need to pause, pause in 'up' position.

✓ Cross your legs, or keep them straight. It is your choice.

✓ Keep your torso as perpendicular to the floor as possible.

Assisted Dips

Beginning Phase: Hands gripping bar, upper body erect, eyes fixed forward. The grip is the same as the standard dip; however, the exercise is accomplished either with a dip assist machine or by a partner clasping the legs or torso (See Figure below).

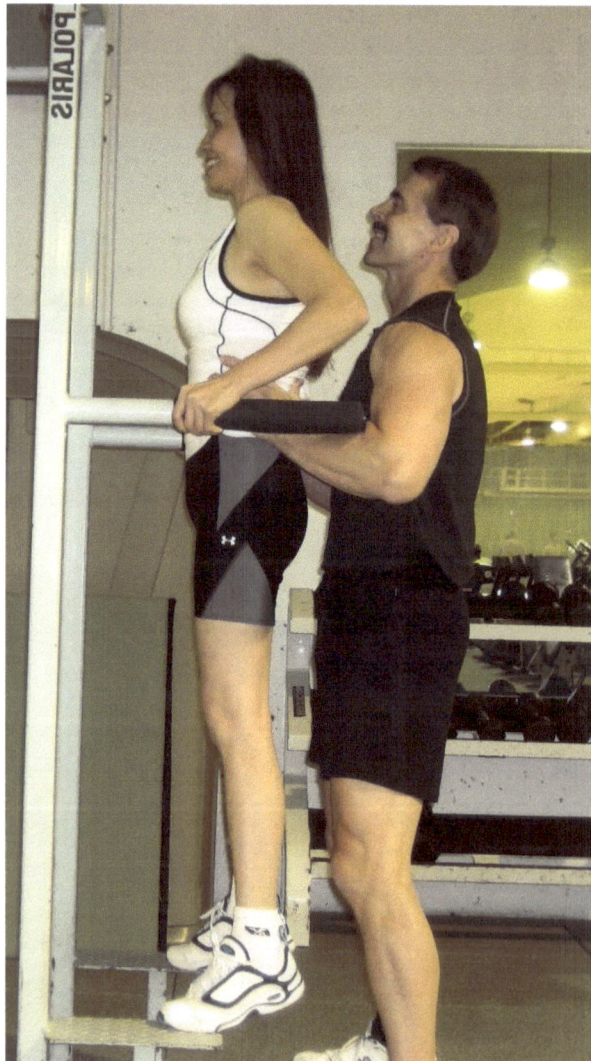

It is critical that good communication is established as the person performing the exercise begins to fatigue. If the assisting partner is holding the legs they must be released in time to prevent injury.

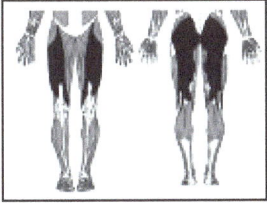

Lunge

Beginning Position: Feet shoulder width apart with toes pointing forward, upper body erect, eyes fixed forward with hands on top of head (Figure below).

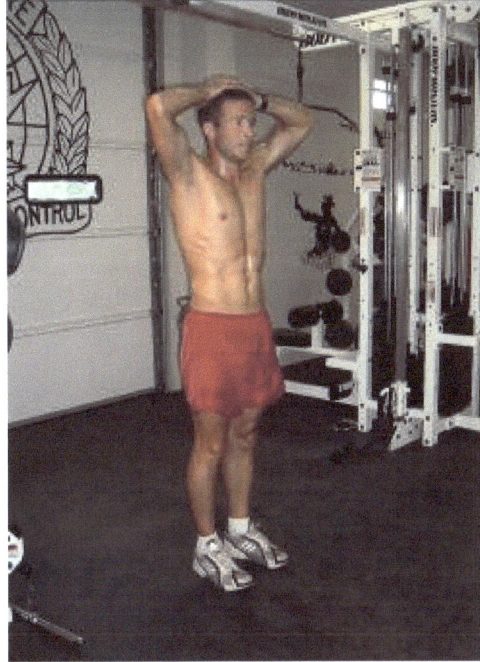

Downward Movement Phase: With the right foot take a large step forward while keeping the left foot in place. Once the right foot is firmly on the floor lower the upper body by bending at the right knee until the upper leg is parallel to the floor. Alternate to the left leg (Figure below).

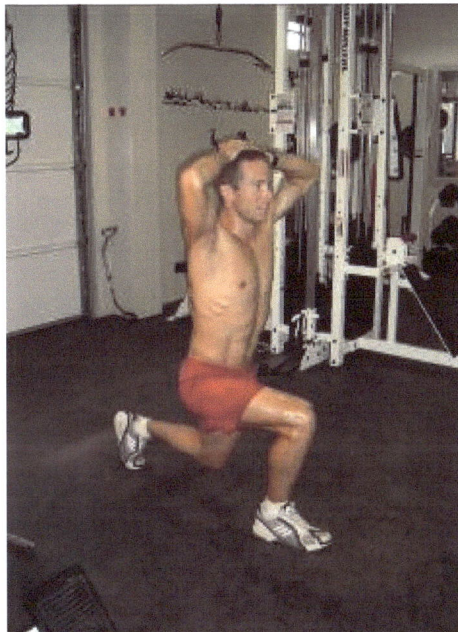

37

Upward Movement Phase: Push with the extended foot in an upward and backward direction in order to raise the body into an erect posture. Maintain a smooth, controlled movement while returning to the position with the legs spread.

❗ TIPS

✓ Perform repetitions as fast as possible without sacrificing form.

✓ The extended foot should be placed far enough forward that the knee does not pass over the front of the foot, but remains directly over the knee.

Alternative to Standard Lunge: Lunges can also be performed with your hands at your hips (Figure below).

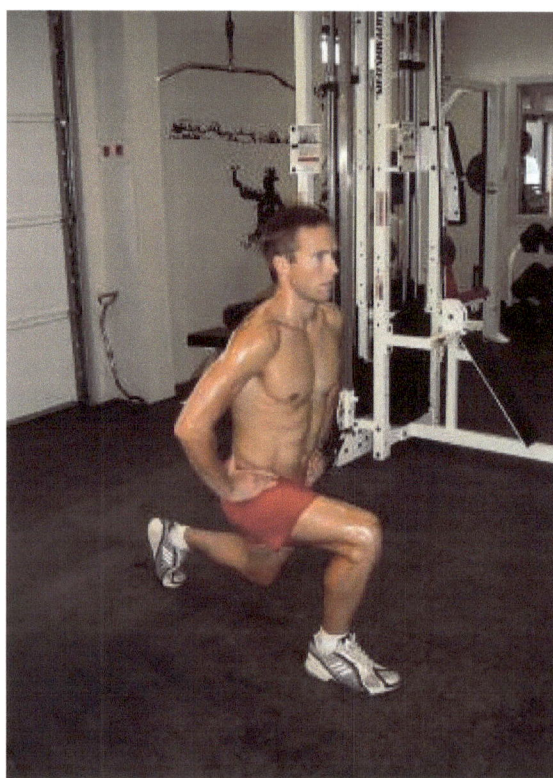

Lunge examples sets

Beginner
6x15 alternating between right and left
45 second time interval

Intermediate
6x25 alternating between right and left
45 second time interval

Hard
6x45 alternating between right and left
60 second time interval

Flutter Kicks

Beginning Phase: Start lying on your back with your hands palms toward the floor and under your gluteals. Raise your feet together approximately 6 inches off the ground. (Figure below).

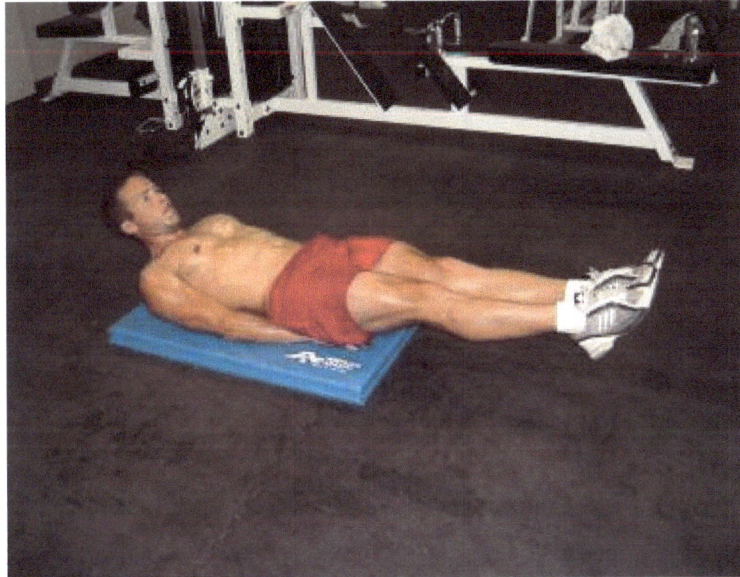

Movement Phase: Bring one leg up to an angle of approximately 45 degrees with reference to the floor while keeping the other leg at 6 inches off the floor. (Figure below).

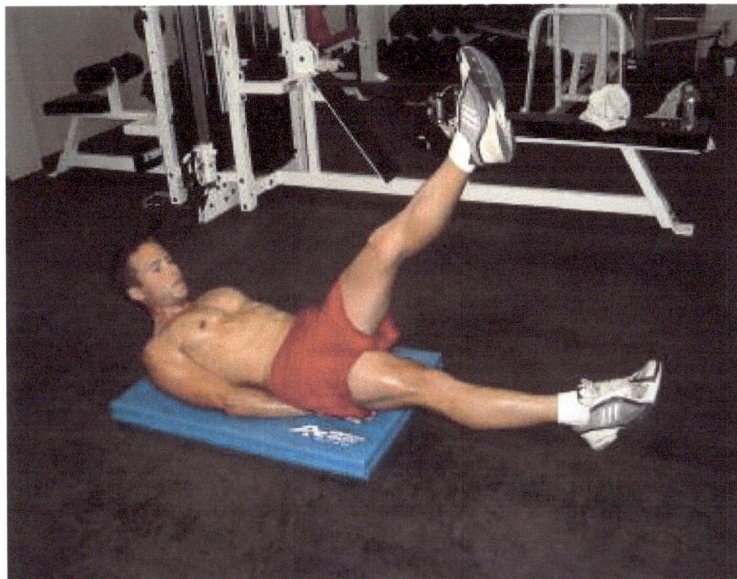

Ending Phase: Alternate legs bringing your opposite leg to the 45 degree angle (Figure below).

! TIPS

Tip: Keep your head up. Keep your legs straight by tightening your abs and flexing your gluteal muscles.

V-Ups

Beginning Phase: Supine with arms extended above your head and legs together and straight and held 6 inches off the ground. (as shown in Figure below).

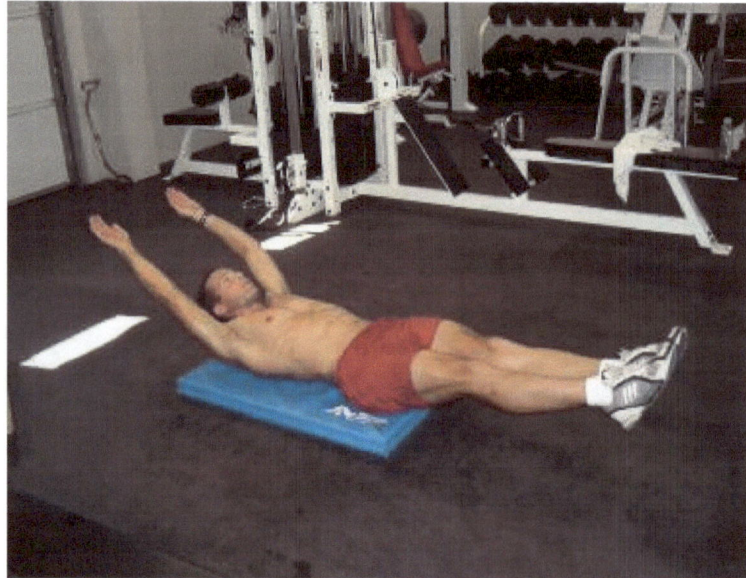

Movement Phase: In synchronous motion bring your hands and feet together, lifting your upper back off the ground. (Figure below).

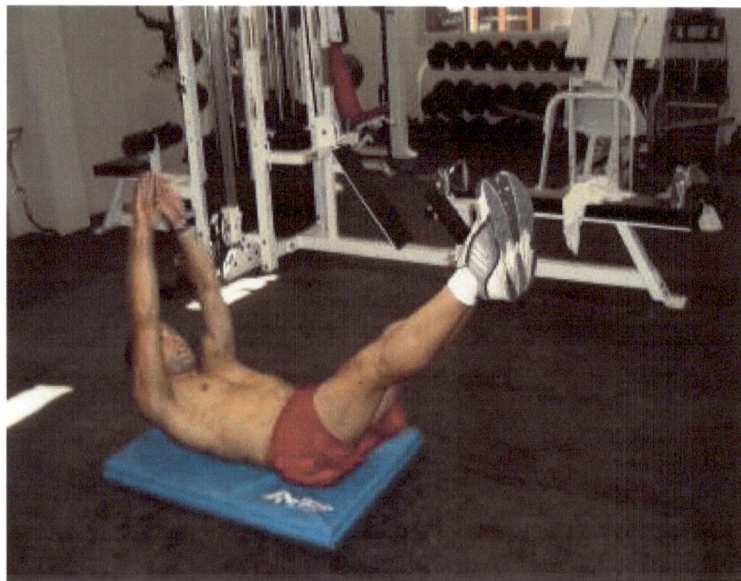

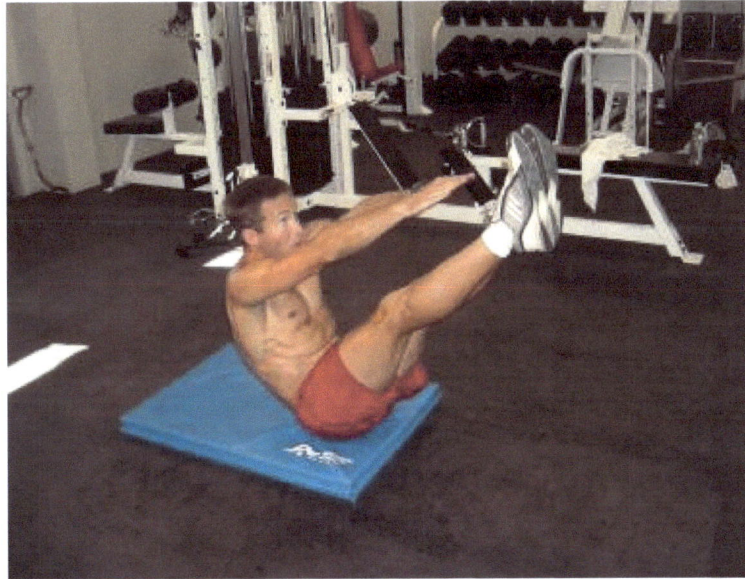

Ending Phase: Slowly bring your upper back down on the mat and lower your legs together until they are again 6 inches off the ground. (Figure below).

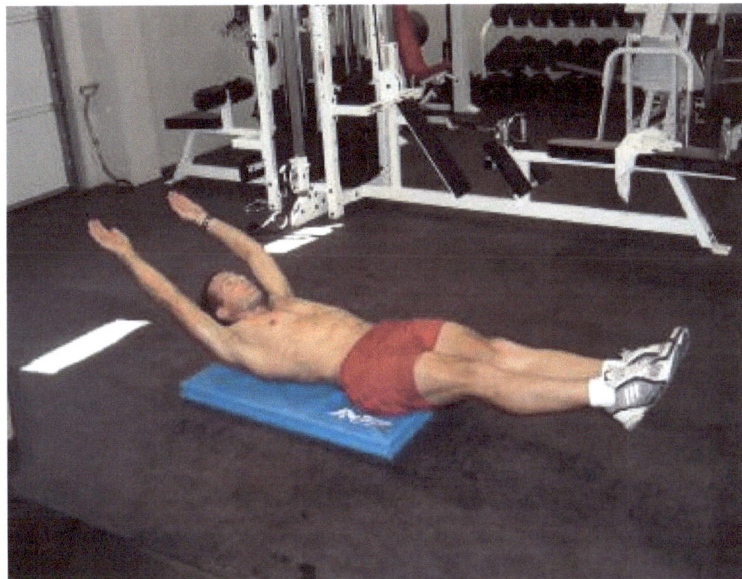

❗ TIPS

Tip: Keep your head up and focus your eyes on an object in front of you. Do not bend your knees or let your back sag. To prevent this; flex your gluteal muscles (butt muscles) and tighten your abs, this will help straighten your knees and back out.

Mad Hubbert's

Beginning Phase: Lying in the supine position with your hands folded on top of your head and feet 6 inches off the floor. (As shown in Figure below).

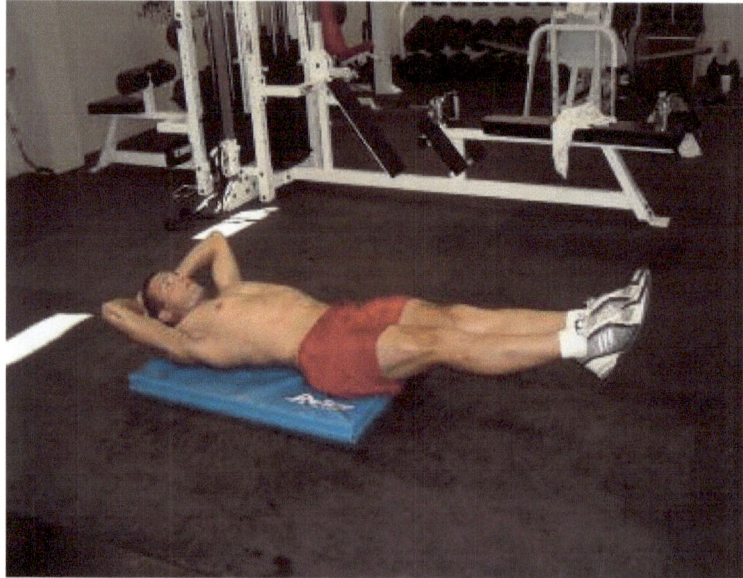

Movement Phase: Bring your elbow to your opposite knee by bringing your lower back off the ground. (Figure below).

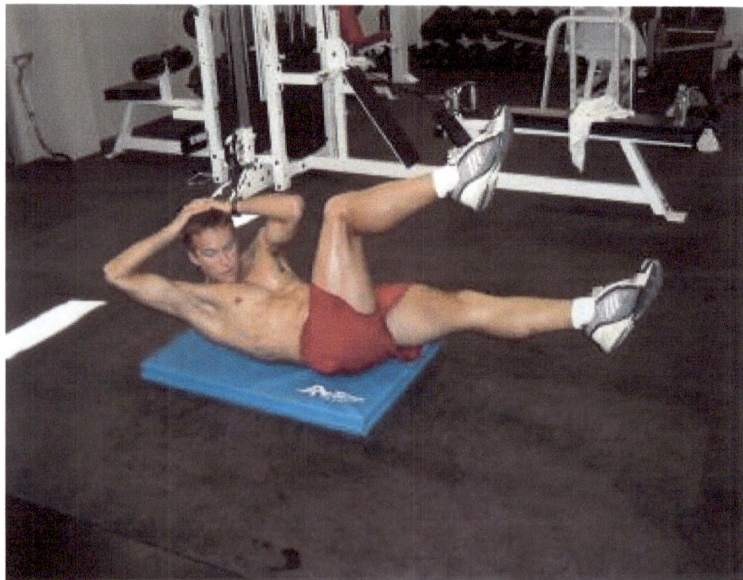

Ending Phase: Slowly bring your back to the ground and your legs to the starting position 6 inches off the ground. (Figure below).

❗ TIPS

Tip: Keep your head up. Do not bend your knees or let your back sag. To prevent this; flex your gluteal muscles (butt muscles) and tighten your abs, this will help straighten your knees and back out.

Hello Dolly's

Beginning Phase: Start lying on your back with your hands palms down under your butt. Raise your feet together approximately 6 inches off the ground as shown in the figure below).

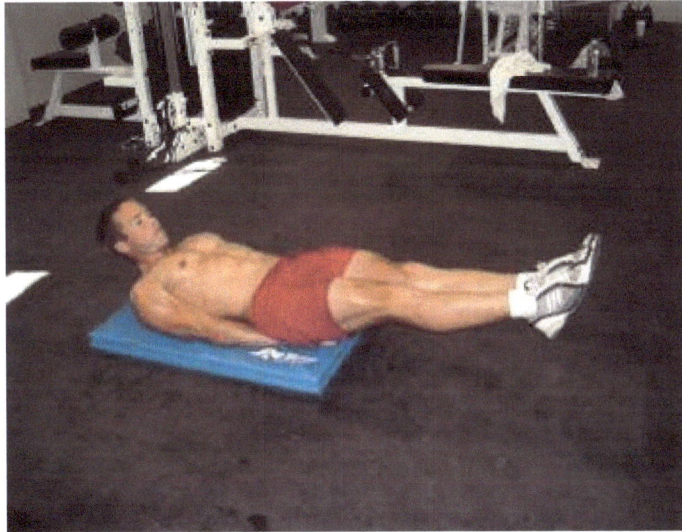

Movement Phase: Separate your legs so they angle away from your body at 45 degrees then bring back together. (Figure below).

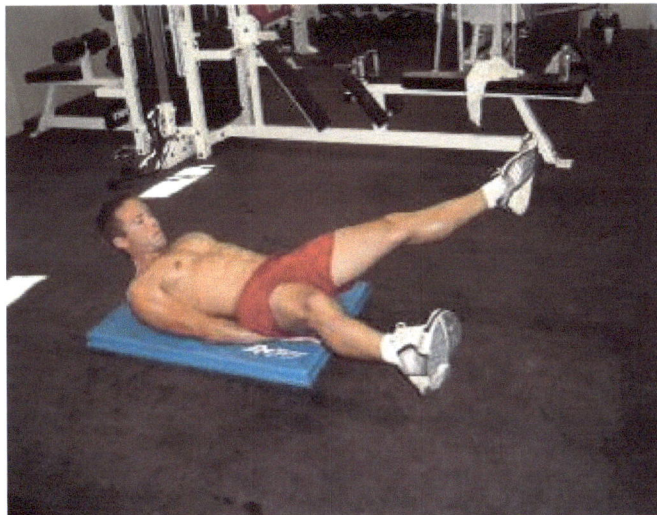

Ending Phase: Bring your legs back together while keeping them 6 inches above the ground (Figure below).

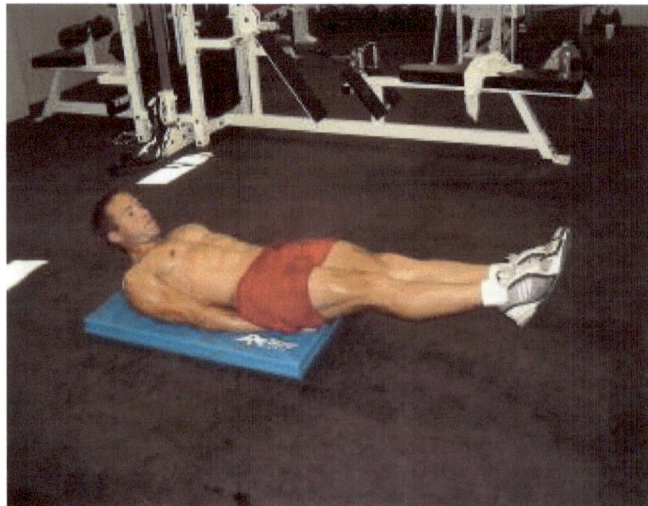

❗ TIPS

Tip: Keep your head up and focus your eyes on an object in front of you. Do not bend your knees or let your back sag. To prevent this; flex your gluteal muscles (butt muscles) and tighten your abs, this will help straighten your knees and back out.

Straight Leg Dead Lifts

Beginning Phase: With your feet shoulder width apart place your hands on your hips. (Figure below).

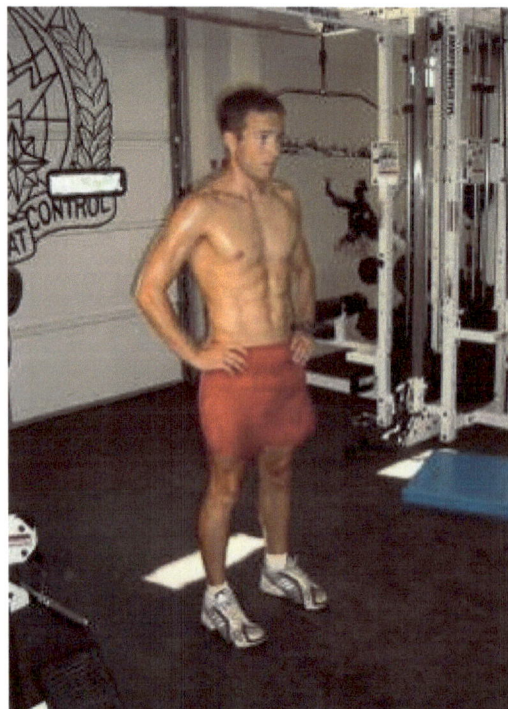

Movement Phase: Lower your upper body by bending at the waist until it is parallel to the floor. (Figure below).

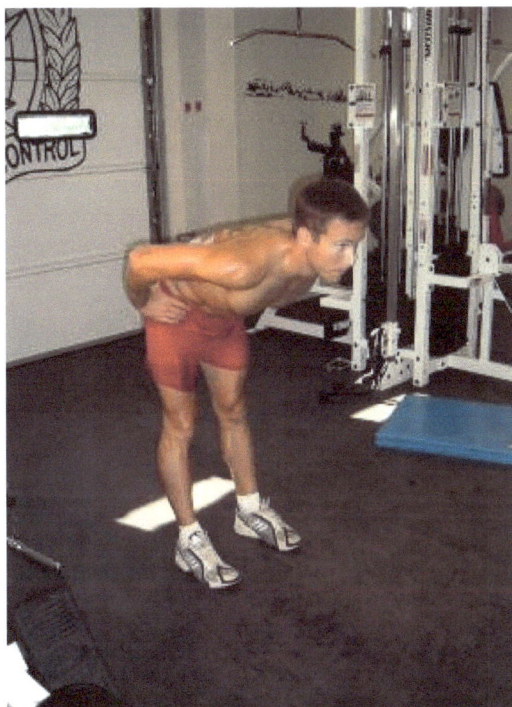

Ending Phase: Bring your upper body back to the erect position (Figure below).

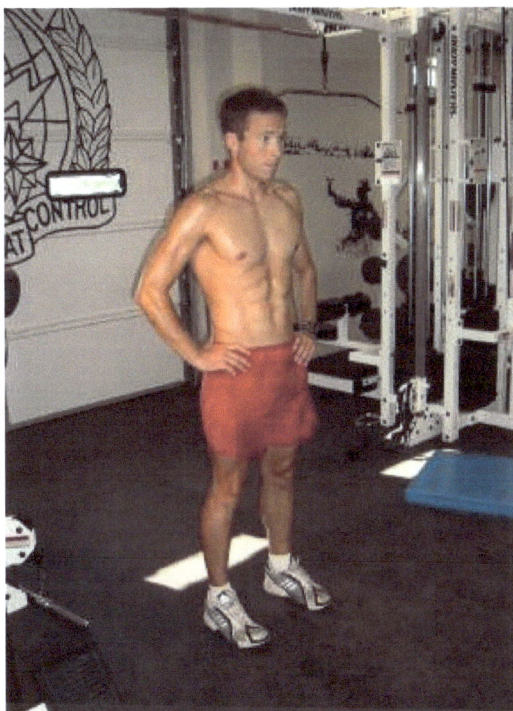

❗ TIPS

Tip: Do not bend your knees. Bend through the waist.

Halo Jumpers

Beginning Phase: Start prone facing the floor with arms extended and shoulder width apart, back flat and feet together (as shown in Figure below).

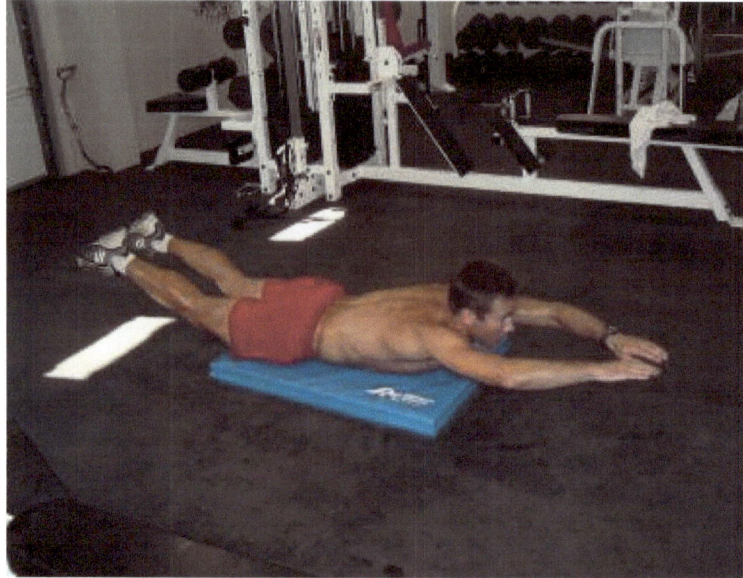

Movement Phase: Arch through the lower back bringing your head, legs, and back up off the floor. (Figure below).

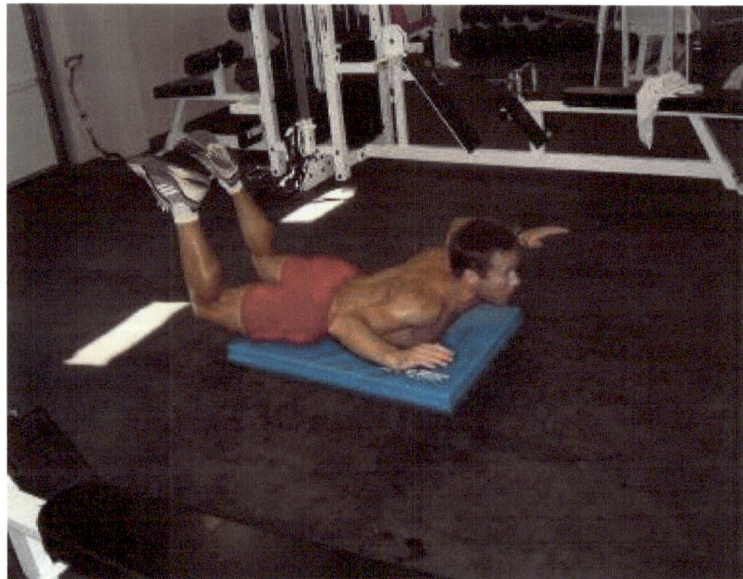

Ending Phase: Slowly bring your arms and legs back to the ground. (Figure below).

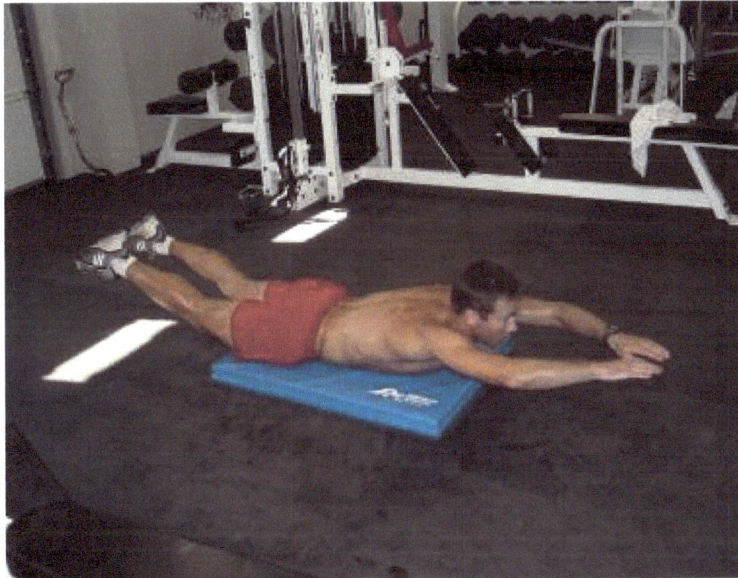

TIPS

Tip: Keep your head up and focus your eyes on an object in front of you. Do not bend your knees or let your back sag. To prevent this; flex your gluteal muscles (butt muscles) and tighten your abs, this will help straighten your knees and back out

---

Superman's

Beginning Phase: Start prone facing the floor with arms extended and shoulder width apart, back flat and feet together (as shown in Figure below).

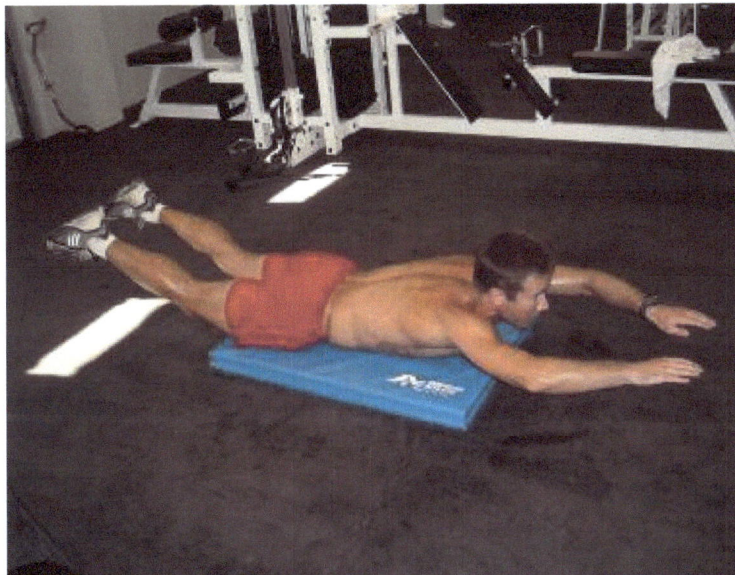

47

Movement Phase: Arch through the lower back bringing your head, legs, and back up off the floor. (Figure below).

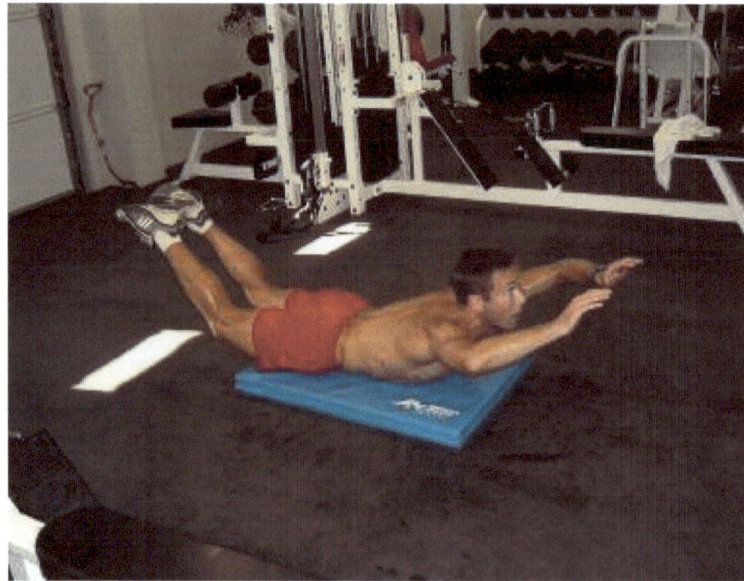

Ending Phase: Slowly bring your arms and legs back to the ground. (Figure below).

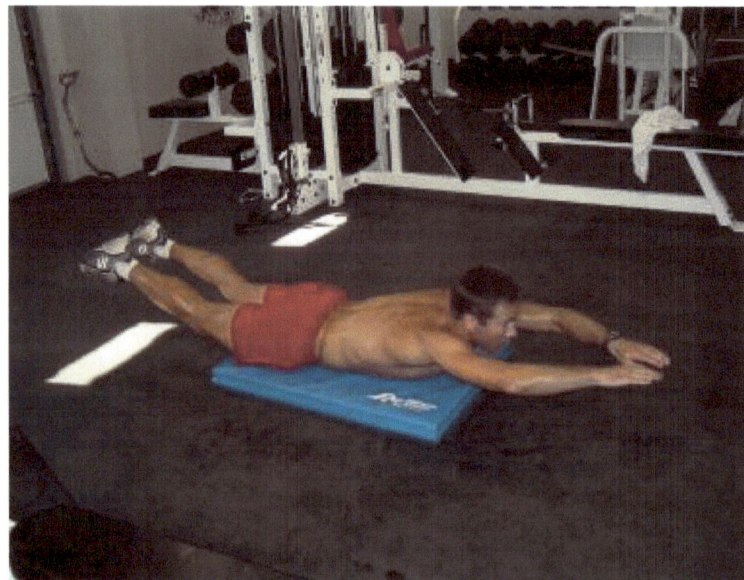

❗ TIPS

Tip: Keep your head up and focus your eyes on an object in front of you. Do not bend your knees or let your back sag. To prevent this; flex your gluteal muscles (butt muscles) and tighten your abs, this will help straighten your knees and back out.

Standard Jumping Jack

Beginning Phase: With feet together and arms at your sides (as shown in Figure below).

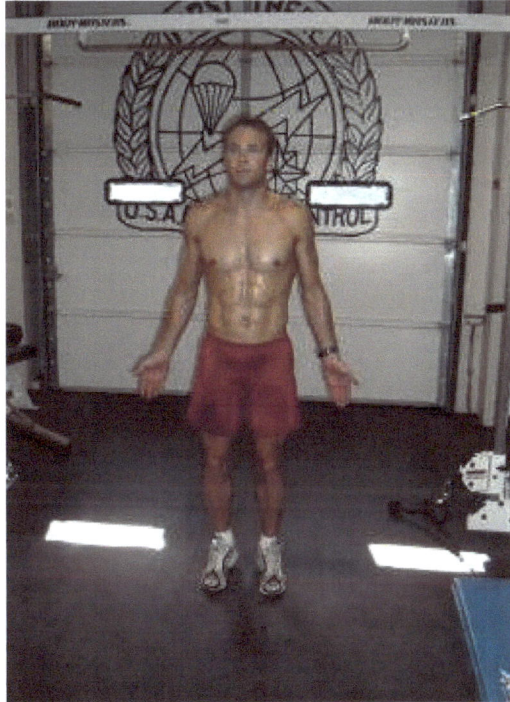

Movement Phase: As your arms leave your sides and meet above your head your feet should separate and to a position slightly wider than your shoulders (Figure below).

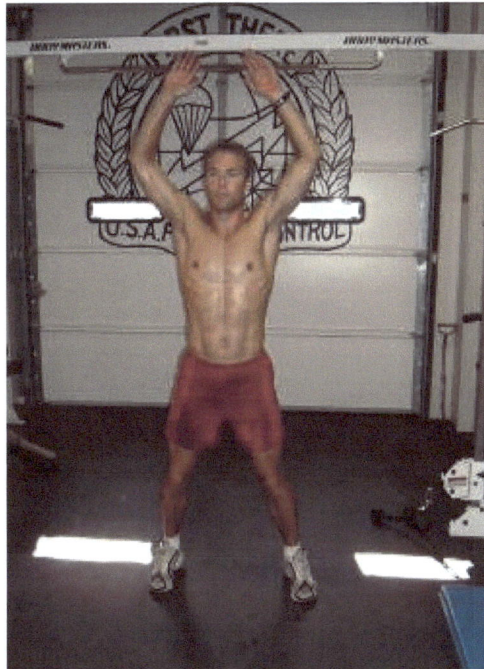

Ending Phase: As you bring your arms down to your sides you simultaneously bring your feet back together (Figure below).

TIPS

Tip: Keep your head up and focus your eyes on an object in front of you..

Air Up

Beginning Phase: Standing and facing forward. Imagine holding a bar in your hands and with your hands near your chest.

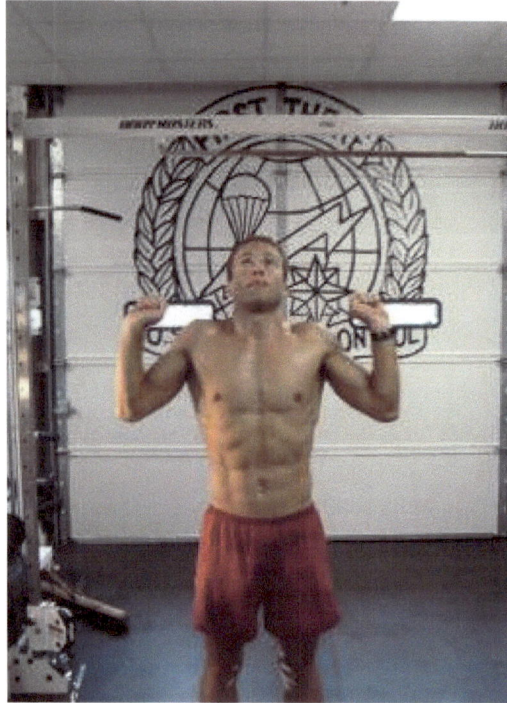

Movement Phase: Press hands above head until elbows are locked out as fast as possible, then without pausing return hands back to starting position.(Figure below).

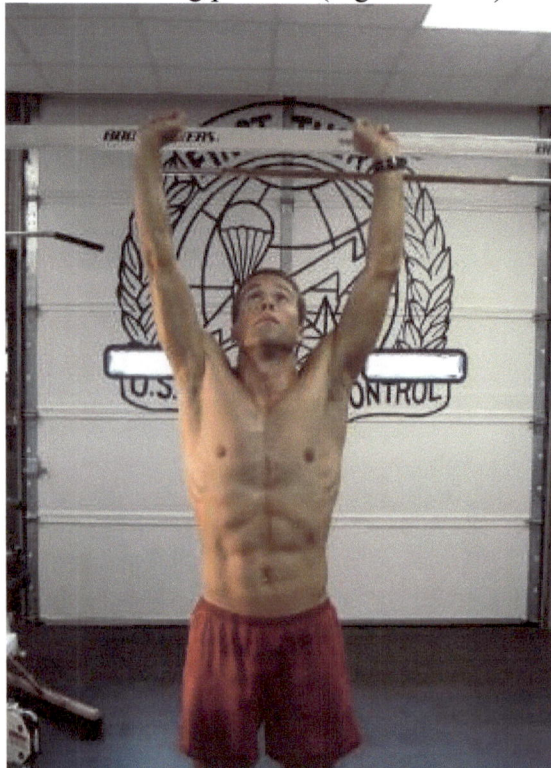

Ending Phase: Bring your hands and arms back to the staring bend position

CHAPTER 4: The Routines

(Reaching your goal in the MINimum amount of time)

We are what we repeatedly do. Excellence, then, is not an act, but a habit.
-Aristotle

IMPORTANT: REMEMBER TO TIME YOURSELF AND FINISH ALL ROUTINES WITHIN A SPECIFIED TIME. These workouts are designed to alternate different muscle groups by changing exercises. As a result a higher heart rate will be maintained. The following are exercise combinations that have yielded outstanding results.

Whole Body Workouts:

A. Beginner Workout: *Time: Complete the following within 30 minutes. You should have 1 minute per exercise.*

Stage One: Easy sets

No	3x	3x	10x	3x	20x
1	Assisted pull-up (regular)	Assisted dip	Beginner push-up	Lunges	Sit-ups
2	Assisted pull-up (wide-grip)	Assisted dip	Beginner push-up	Lunges	Sit-ups
3	Assisted chin-up	Assisted dip	Beginner push-up	Lunges	Sit-ups
4	Assisted close-grip pull-up	Assisted dip	Beginner push-up	Lunges	Sit-ups
5	Assisted cross grip pull-up	Assisted dip	Beginner push-up	Lunges	Sit-ups
6	Assisted (alternate) cross grip pull-up	Assisted dip	Beginner push-up	Lunges	Sit-ups

*Lunges refer to the number per leg (e.g. 3 lunges means 3 per leg or a total of 6).

Stage Two: Intermediate sets

No	6x	6x	15x	6x	30x
7	Assisted pull-up (regular)	Assisted dip	Beginner push-up	Lunges	Sit-ups
8	Assisted pull-up (wide-grip)	Assisted dip	Beginner push-up	Lunges	Sit-ups
9	Assisted chin-up	Assisted dip	Beginner push-up	Lunges	Sit-ups
10	Assisted close-grip pull-up	Assisted dip	Beginner push-up	Lunges	Sit-ups
11	Assisted cross grip pull-up	Assisted dip	Beginner push-up	Lunges	Sit-ups
12	Assisted (alternate) cross grip pull-up	Assisted dip	Beginner push-up	Lunges	Sit-ups

Stage Three: Hard sets

No	9x	9x	20x	9x	40x
13	Assisted pull-up (regular)	Assisted dip	Beginner push-up	Lunges	Sit-ups
14	Assisted pull-up (wide-grip)	Assisted dip	Beginner push-up	Lunges	Sit-ups
15	Assisted chin-up	Assisted dip	Beginner push-up	Lunges	Sit-ups
16	Assisted close-grip pull-up	Assisted dip	Beginner push-up	Lunges	Sit-ups
17	Assisted cross grip pull-up	Assisted dip	Beginner push-up	Lunges	Sit-ups
18	Assisted (alternate) cross grip pull-up	Assisted dip	Beginner push-up	Lunges	Sit-ups

B. Intermediate Routine:

Time: Complete the following within 30 minutes. You should have 1 minute per exercise.

Stage One: Easy sets

No	3x	3x	10x	3x	25x
1	pull-up (regular)	dip	push-up	Lunges	Sit-ups
2	pull-up (wide-grip)	dip	push-up	Lunges	Sit-ups
3	chin-up	dip	push-up	Lunges	Sit-ups
4	close-grip pull-up	dip	Beginner push-up	Lunges	Sit-ups
5	cross grip pull-up	dip	Beginner push-up	Lunges	Sit-ups
6	(alternate) cross grip pull-up	dip	Beginner push-up	Lunges	Sit-ups

*Lunges refer to the number per leg (e.g. 3 lunges means 3 per leg or a total of 6).

Stage Two: Intermediate sets

No	5x	5x	15x	5x	35x
7	pull-up (regular)	dip	push-up	Lunges	Sit-ups
8	pull-up (wide-grip)	dip	push-up	Lunges	Sit-ups
9	chin-up	dip	push-up	Lunges	Sit-ups
10	close-grip pull-up	dip	push-up	Lunges	Sit-ups
11	cross grip pull-up	dip	push-up	Lunges	Sit-ups
12	(alternate) cross grip pull-up	dip	push-up	Lunges	Sit-ups

Stage Three: Hard sets

No	10x	10x	20x	10x	45x
13	pull-up (regular)	dip	push-up	Lunges	Sit-ups
14	pull-up (wide-grip)	dip	push-up	Lunges	Sit-ups
15	chin-up	dip	push-up	Lunges	Sit-ups
16	close-grip pull-up	dip	push-up	Lunges	Sit-ups
17	cross grip pull-up	dip	push-up	Lunges	Sit-ups
18	(alternate) cross grip pull-up	dip	push-up	Lunges	Sit-ups

C. Advanced Routine: For the serious athlete
Time: Complete the following within 30 minutes. You should have 1 minute per exercise.

Stage One: Easy sets

No	5x	5x	25x	5x	30x
1	pull-up (regular)	dip	push-up	Lunges	Sit-ups
2	pull-up (wide-grip)	dip	push-up	Lunges	Sit-ups
3	chin-up	dip	push-up	Lunges	Sit-ups
4	close-grip pull-up	dip	Beginner push-up	Lunges	Sit-ups
5	cross grip pull-up	dip	Beginner push-up	Lunges	Sit-ups
6	(alternate) cross grip pull-up	dip	Beginner push-up	Lunges	Sit-ups

Stage Two: Intermediate sets

No	10x	10x	30x	10x	40x
7	pull-up (regular)	dip	push-up	Lunges	Sit-ups
8	pull-up (wide-grip)	dip	push-up	Lunges	Sit-ups
9	chin-up	dip	push-up	Lunges	Sit-ups
10	close-grip pull-up	dip	push-up	Lunges	Sit-ups
11	cross grip pull-up	dip	push-up	Lunges	Sit-ups
12	(alternate) cross grip pull-up	dip	push-up	Lunges	Sit-ups

Stage Three: Hard sets

No	15x	20x	35x	15x	50x
13	pull-up (regular)	dip	push-up	Lunges	Sit-ups
14	pull-up (wide-grip)	dip	push-up	Lunges	Sit-ups
15	chin-up	dip	push-up	Lunges	Sit-ups
16	close-grip pull-up	dip	push-up	Lunges	Sit-ups
17	cross grip pull-up	dip	push-up	Lunges	Sit-ups
18	(alternate) cross grip pull-up	dip	push-up	Lunges	Sit-ups

Try the following alternate Routines to be used 1-2 times per month for variety:

Interval sets

Easy:
 10x2 pull-ups
10x10 pushups
10x10 sit-ups
10x5 dips
10x10 lunges

Intermediate:

10x5 pull-ups
10x15 push-ups
10x15 sit-ups
10x8 dips
10x15 lunges

Advanced:

10x10 pull-ups
10x25 push-ups
10x25 sit-ups
10x15 dips
10x20 lunges

Pyramid sets

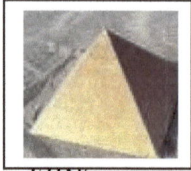

Almost any exercise can have a pyramid workout applied to it. The goal is to start out slowly at a warm-up level then max out at the peak of the workout and work back down as a warm-down. For example, pull-ups, push-ups, and sit-ups can be alternated up to a desired number up to a maximum repetition.

Easy:
Pull-ups: 2,3,4,5,4,3,2
Sit-ups: 10,15,20,25,20,15,10
Dips: 4,6,8,10,8,6,4
Pushups: 5,10,15,20,15,10,5
Lunges: 5,10,15,20,15,10,5

Intermediate:
Pull-ups: 4,6,8,10,8,6,4
Sit-ups: 20,30,40,50,40,30,20
Dips: 5,10,15,20,15,10,5
Pushups: 10,20,30,40,30,20,10
Lunges: 10,20,30,40,30,20,10

Advanced:
Pull-ups: 5,10,15,20,15,10,5
Sit-ups: 25,50,75,100,75,50,25
Dips: 10,20,30,40,30,20,10
Pushups: 20,40,60,80,60,40,20
Lunges: 20,40,60,80,60,40,20

Weight-Assisted Routines: As the routines become easier, one can add additional weight to your body's own weight. This involves using a weight supportive belt, and a chain to suspend weights from your waist (Figure below)

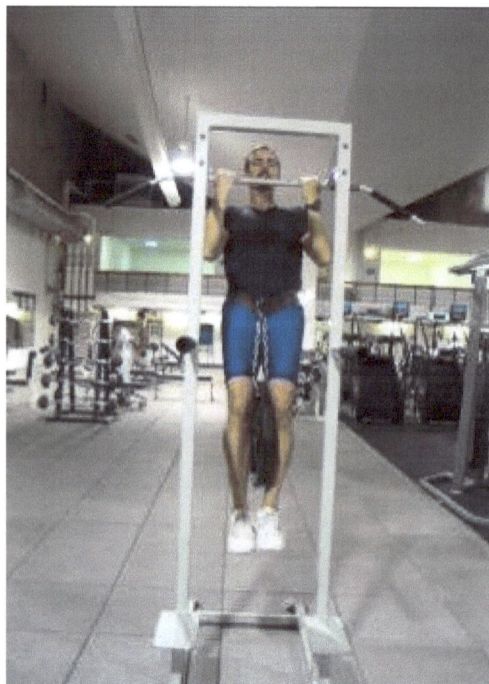

Upper Body Only Routines

A. Beginners Routine: Almost anyone can do these routines. If you are weaker in the arms and shoulders, begin as follows:

Time: Complete each of the following stages within 18 minutes. You should have 1 minute per exercise.

Assisted pull-ups: Try doing and completing sets with help before proceeding to independent sets.

Stage one: Beginner sets

    1 assisted pull-up (regular) - 3 assisted dips - 5 beginner push-ups
    2 assisted pull-ups (wide-grip) - 6 assisted dips - 10 beginner push-ups
    3 assisted chin-ups - 3 assisted dips- 9 beginner -15push-ups
    3 assisted close-grip pull-ups - 9 assisted dips - 15 beginner push-ups
    2 assisted cross-grip pull-ups - 6 assisted dips - 10 beginner push-ups
    1 assisted (alternate) cross-grip pull-ups - 3 assisted dips- 5 beginner push-ups

Stage Two: Intermediate sets

    1 assisted pull-ups (regular) - 3 assisted dips - 10 beginner push-ups
    2 assisted pull-ups (wide-grip) - 3 assisted dips - 10 beginner push-ups
    3 assisted chin-ups - 3 assisted dips - 10 beginner push-ups
    4 assisted close-grip pull-ups - 3 assisted dips - 10 beginner push-ups
    5 assisted cross-grip pull-ups - 3 assisted dips - 10 beginner push-ups
    6 assisted cross-grip pull-ups - 3 assisted dips- 10 beginner push-ups

Stage Three: Advanced sets

    6 assisted pull-ups (regular) - 3 assisted dips - 10 beginner push-ups
    5 assisted pull-ups (wide-grip) - 3 assisted dips - 10 beginner push-ups
    4 assisted chin-ups - 3 assisted dips - 10 beginner push-ups
    3 assisted close-grip pull-ups- 3 assisted dips - 10 beginner push-ups
    2 assisted cross-grip pull-ups- 3 assisted dips - 10 beginner push-ups
    1 assisted cross-grip pull-ups - 3 assisted dips - 10 beginner push-ups

B. Intermediate Routine:

Time: Complete each of the following stages within 18 minutes. You should have 1 minute per exercise.

Stage one: Beginner sets

    3 pull-ups (regular) - 3 dips- 10 push-ups
    3 pull-ups (wide-grip) - 3 dips - 10 push-ups
    3 chin-ups - 3 dips - 10 push-ups
    3 close-grip pull-ups - 3 dips - 10 push-ups
    3 cross-grip pull-ups- 3 dips - 10 push-ups
    3 cross-grip pull-ups - 3 dips - 10 push-ups

Stage Two: Intermediate sets

    5 pull-ups (regular) - 5 dips - 10 push-ups
    5 pull-ups (wide-grip) - 5 dips - 10 push-ups
    5 chin-ups - 5 dips- 10 push-ups
    5 close-grip pull-ups- 5 dips - 10 push-ups
    5 cross-grip pull-ups- 5 dips - 10 push-ups
    5 cross-grip pull-ups - 5 dips - 10 push-ups

Stage Three: Hard set

    10 pull-ups (regular) - 10 dips - 10 push-ups
    10 pull-ups (wide-grip) - 10 dips- 10 push-ups
    10 chin-ups - 10 dips - 10 push-ups
    10 close-grip pull-ups - 10 dips - 10 push-ups
    10 cross-grip pull-ups - 10 dips- 10 push-ups
    10 cross-grip pull-ups - 10 dips- 10 push-ups

C. Advanced Routine: For the serious athlete

Time: Complete each of the following within 18 minutes. You should have 1 minute per exercise.

Stage one: Beginner sets

    5 pull-ups (regular) - 5 dips - 25 push-ups
    5 pull-ups (wide-grip) - 5 dips - 25 push-ups
    5 chin-ups - 5 dips - 25 push-ups
    5 close-grip pull-ups - 5 dips - 25 push-ups
    5 cross-grip pull-ups- 5 dips - 25 push-ups
    5 cross-grip pull-ups - 5 dips - 25 push-ups

Stage Two: Intermediate sets

    10 pull-ups (regular) - 10 dips- 25 push-ups
    10 pull-ups (wide-grip) - 10 dips - 25 push-ups
    10 chin-ups - 10 dips - 25 push-ups
    10 close-grip pull-ups - 10 dips - 25 push-ups
    10 cross-grip pull-ups - 10 dips - 25 push-ups
    10 cross-grip pull-ups - 10 dips- 25 push-ups

Stage Three: Hard sets

    15 pull-ups (regular) - 15 dips - 25 push-ups
    15 pull-ups (wide-grip) - 15 dips - 25 push-ups
    15 chin-ups - 15 dips - 25 push-ups
    15 close-grip pull-ups - 15 dips - 25 push-ups
    15 cross-grip pull-ups - 15 dips - 25 push-ups
    15 cross-grip pull-ups - 15 dips - 25 push-ups

Additional Suggested Workouts:

A. Easy:

10x5 pullups
10x15 pushups
10x10 dips
10x15 situps
10x15 lunges

Total time: 50 minutes
Each round of exercises is completed in 5 minutes.
1 minute per set

B. Intermediate:

10x10 pullups
10x25 pushups
10x15 dips
10x25 situps
10x15 lunges

Total time: 50 minutes
Each round of exercises is completed in 5 minutes.
1 minute per set

C. Advanced:

10x20 pullups
10x50 pushups
10x30 dips
10x50 situps
10x50 lunges

Total time: 50 minutes
Each round of exercises is completed in 5 minutes.
1 minute per set

CHAPTER 5: How Should I Eat to Perform at My Best?
(Using nutrition to your advantage)

"To eat is a necessity, but to eat intelligently is an art."
- *La Rochefoucauld*

Eating Basics: Many people fail to make nutrition an integral part of their training program. They accomplish their training but miss an important link - fueling well. You must incorporate optimal eating into a busy lifestyle. You should fuel at your best, so you can train at your best and compete at your best. Eating properly is essential to providing the energy/nutrients needed to improve your well-being. While nutrition alone cannot turn you into an Olympic athlete, with good nutritional habits you can reach your full potential. Sound nutritional habits are essential for you to perform at your best, while at the same time providing adequate nutrients for growth, repair and tissue maintenance. While this chapter is not intended as an exhaustive text on sports nutrition, it attempts to present basic principles and give examples of proper nutrition to facilitate exercise performance.

Activity Level: An exact estimation of daily caloric intake in any given individual is difficult due to genetics, medical illnesses, lifestyles, and other variables. Higher caloric requirements are an outcome of all athletic endeavors. Nutrition may be manipulated at nearly every level of activity to improve performance. To begin to understand what your nutritional needs will be when undertaking a physically demanding exercise routine, it is important to classify your activity level with regards to the general population.

- Training for general health & fitness:
    0.5 to 1 hour, 3-5 times per week
- Recreational athlete:
    1-1.5 hours, 3-5 times per week
- Well-trained athlete:
    1.5-3 hours, 5-7 times per week
- Elite/World Class athlete:
    2-6 hours, 6-10 times per week

General Principles: Regardless of your fitness levels, you should adopt some of these basic healthy eating habits.

- If you do not feel hungry, don't eat. You can avoid several hundred calories per day by only eating when you have the urge to eat, versus eating out of boredom, eating social gatherings, or eating because it is "time" to eat.
- Do not eat while watching TV or a movie or while driving. When you do eat, focus on the food and enjoy it rather than mindlessly placing food into your mouth and not noticing your body's signals of feeling full.
- Never eat until you are full. Always stop eating when you are satisfied and no longer hungry. Avoid that 'overstuffed' feeling. It is better to leave the table knowing you could eat more than to force down those last few bites.
- Do not let the scale dictate who you are. Put your bathroom scale in the corner and forget about it for a couple weeks. Monitor yourself by how your clothes are fitting. Are your clothes fitting tightly or loosely? Do you now need a belt to hold your pants up, or have your belt tightened a notch? How do your arms and shoulders fit in your shirts? How about your chest circumference? Let how you feel help you eat properly.

- o If you absolutely cannot give up the scale then be certain to weigh yourself at the same time everyday. The preferred time is first thing in the morning. Body weight can fluctuate throughout the day depending on the time of day and hydration status. A rapid change in weight is most likely due to hydration status. A woman's menstrual cycle can also cause fluctuation of body weight throughout the month. Weight is an inherently poor measure of how your fitness status is progressing, yet one that many have fixated upon. Ignore weight and measure yourself through other means.
- Drink 2 full glasses of water before every meal and every time you feel hungry. Then reevaluate how hungry you really are. Did the water fill you up, or does your body really need food?
- Eat slowly. After you have drunk two full glasses of water and still feel hungry go ahead and eat. Chew each bite completely swallow and count to 10 before your next bite. Are you satisfied after a couple of bites? If you are eating a snack, could you walk away now and come back in an hour to finish the snack? Small amounts of food spaced throughout the day are healthier than large food boluses at any one given time.
- Before purchasing packaged foods and supplements read the label. All packaged food products are required by the Food and Drug Administration (FDA) to have labels with information containing serving size, calories, and key nutrients. Pay particular attention to how many servings are in the package. The calories and nutrients listed apply to one serving.
- If you are full, do not "clean your plate." It has been ingrained in us since we were children and our parents told us to "clean our plates before leaving the table." Well, your parents were wrong. This is a bad habit many require you to continue eating to the point of discomfort. If you find yourself doing this make a conscious effort to stop.

Your Weight in Kilograms: Since the metric system is universal, use this system for quantifying weight. Every packaged item of food you buy is also on the metric system. Thus it is important to find out your weight in kilograms so we can find the proper number of grams you should be consuming. The exact way to determine your weight in kilograms is to divide your weight in pounds by 2.2. An easy way to do this is divide your weight in pounds by 2, then subtract 10% (e.g. 100 pounds / 2 =50, 10% of 50=5, 50 - 5=45 kg).

- 2.2 Pounds = 1 Kilogram
    - 99 lbs = 45kg
    - 110 lbs = 50 kg
    - 121 lbs = 55 kg
    - 132 lbs = 60 kg
    - 143 lbs = 65 kg
    - 154 lbs = 70 kg
    - 165 lbs = 75 kg
    - 176 lbs = 80 kg
    - 187 lbs = 85 kg
    - 198 lbs = 90 kg
    - 209 lbs = 95 kg
    - 220 lbs = 100 kg
    - 231 lbs = 105 kg
    - 242 lbs = 110 kg
    - 253 lbs = 115 kg

262 lbs = 120 kg

Energy Needs: Once you have determined your weight in kilograms and have been honest with how you classify yourself, you are now able to more accurately find the calorie range you should attempt to maintain. One nutritional calorie = 1 kcal of energy. The typical daily caloric needs is somewhere between 30 to 40 kcal/kg body weight/day. However an elite individual may require 45 to 50 kcal/kg body weight/day and may need more during serious training (>50 kcal/kg body weight/day). MAXimize the MINimum incorporates strength training to obtain high levels of fat-free mass. In circumstances in which an increase in lean body mass is the goal, energy intake must be sufficient to meet the needs for muscle growth.

If your activity ranges from sedentary to a recreational athlete, your goals can be achieved through smart food choices and training. Even with well-trained or elite athletes, supplementation does not guarantee success.

Table for Calculating Caloric Requirements

Activity Level	Calculation
Recreational Athlete	Weight (kg) x 30
Well-Trained	Weight (kg) x 40
Elite/World Class	Weight (kg) x 45

Why Not Measure Food Composition as a Percentage of Diet: As you may notice in this chapter, grams are used instead of a percentage (%) of diet. It is less likely to inadvertently cause a dietary deficiency by recommending amounts of carbohydrate, protein, and fat. Dietary or energy deficiency can manifest as weight loss, inability to adapt to training, diminished performance, muscle soreness, respiratory infections, and symptoms characteristic of overtraining such as insomnia, lack of training progression, weakened immune system, decrease in performance, and irritability.

Macronutrients: The three basic food components that are necessary in large quantities are:
- Carbohydrates
- Proteins
- Fats

These three substances make up the bulk of the required nutrients for performance and everyday bodily functions. The basic requirements are the same for active and sedentary people, However as activity level increases greater dietary intake is required.

Carbohydrates: They are the most important energy source for muscle training and are stored in the liver and to a lesser degree muscle in the form of glycogen and in the blood as glucose. Carbohydrates supply most of the energy for working muscle. Prolonged exercise will deplete the body of its glycogen stores and lead to fatigue with inability to continue the exercise. Adequate amounts of carbohydrates are consumed to maintain glycogen stores and maintain energy levels. The typical American diet contains suboptimal amounts of carbohydrates and too much protein and fats.

Carbohydrates are the most important energy source for your workout. Complex carbohydrates such as fruits, vegetables, and unprocessed whole grains should make up the majority of your diet. Simple carbohydrates like table sugar should be ingested in limited quantities.

The Glycemic Index: The Glycemic Index (GI) ranks carbohydrate-rich foods based on their rate of digestion and absorption. Moderate to high GI foods can efficiently deliver carbohydrate to the body during exercise and recovery. The athletic snack industry has begun to tailor their product for athletic use (e.g. drinks, gels, bars).

However, when outside of the peri-workout time period the bulk of the carbohydrate consumed in the overall diet should have a low glycemic index.

Glycemic Index of Common Foods
(55-100+ is considered high)

Maltose	105
Glucose	100
White Bread	95
Baked Potatoes	95
Carrots (cooked)	85
Rice Cakes	80
Honey	75
Refined Sugar	75
Corn (cooked)	75
Puffed Wheat	75
Cornflakes	75
White Rice	70
Shredded Wheat	70
Millet	70
Raisins (seedless)	65
Pasta	65
Bananas	60
Spaghetti	60
Rye or Sourdough bread	55
Wild Rice	55
Brown Rice	55
Popcorn	55
Kiwi, Grape, Mango	50
Whole Grain Pasta	45
Plum, Apple, Orange	40
Apricot (dried)	30
Milk	20
Tomatoes	15
Green Vegetables	0-15

Protein: Proteins are the building blocks for muscle, hair, and nails and are intimately involved in energy production, muscle contraction, and structural roles.

Contrary to popular belief weight lifting alone does not increase the need for protein in the diet. Over the years many athletes seeking to increase body mass have ingested massive quantities of protein and amino acid supplements. At the present time there is no strong evidence suggesting that protein supplements are needed for optimal muscle growth or muscle strength. However, athletes who participate in endurance training may require more protein than sedentary individuals. The typical American diet contains more than enough total energy (calories) as protein. Extra intake of protein in the form of protein drinks and pills is usually unnecessary. Although excess protein in healthy individuals has not been shown to have any deleterious effects, just like all other excess calories, additional protein in the diet will be stored as body fat. Although most people eat more protein than necessary, good choices for protein intake in a regular American diet can be found in high quality beef, chicken, fish, low fat dairy, beans, and eggs.

Protein is most critical during the post-workout period. It provides amino acids for the building and repair of muscle tissue. In general, you should consume a mixed meal providing carbohydrates and protein soon after a strenuous competition or training session. The ideal ratio of carbohydrate to protein is 4 grams carbohydrate to 1 gram protein.

Fat: Fat is essential to every diet, but should be consumed in modest amounts. Fat is important as the major form of stored energy. It provides energy in prolonged periods without food and serves as your body's basal energy source. It is also important to insulate and protect organs. Your diet should be low, but not devoid of fat. Prior to a workout, during a workout, or immediately after a workout, meals and snacks should be relatively low in fat and fiber to facilitate stomach emptying prior to activity.

Fats provide over twice the amount of calories per gram when compared to carbohydrates and protein. It is important to know that not all fats are created equal. Fats differ in their type and saturation. The food package label will list the number of calories from fat, as well as the amount of saturated and unsaturated (trans) fats. Trans fats have been linked to coronary artery disease (plaque build up in heart arteries), and cerebral vascular accidents (strokes). Trans fat has the double the effect of elevating blood lipid levels (amount of fat in bloodstream). There is really no reason to consume trans fat and some countries (e.g., Denmark) have imposed a ban on trans fats. Consumers should take advantage of the new labeling regulations and select products that contain low levels of trans and saturated fats. An easy way to tell if an oil has a high amount of trans fat is if it is a solid at room temperature. Examples include, butter, shortening, margarines, baked goods, snack foods, fried foods, salad dressings, and processed foods.

One particularly important type of fat is omega-3 fatty acids. Omega-3 fats are ideal, owing to the fact that they modulate the inflammatory response. Several studies have shown that omega-3 fatty acids may decrease inflammation in sufferers of rheumatoid arthritis. There is also a possible role for them in athletes by helping to decrease training injuries and soreness. Also, recent literature has supported their use as a secondary preventive measure in reduction of total mortality, death from coronary heart disease, and sudden death. They are found in highest concentrations in fish. Other foods with omega-3 fats include soybean, canola, and flax seed oil.

Daily Nutritional Needs

Activity Level	General Health & Fitness	Recreational	Well-Trained	Elite
Carbohydrates	5-8 g/kg/day	5-8 g/kg/day	8-10 g/kg/day	8-10 g/kg/day
Protein	1-1.5 g/kg/day	1-1.5 g/kg/day	1.5-2.0 g/kg/day	1.5-2.0 g/kg/day
Fat	0.5-1 g/kg/day	0.5-1 g/kg/day	0.5-1 g/kg/day	0.5-1 g/kg/day

Micronutrients: These are substances that are necessary in small quantities and aid in regulation of many metabolic processes. The two basic components are:

- Vitamins
- Minerals

Vitamins and minerals play very important roles in maintaining efficient and effective energy transfers throughout the body. In nearly all circumstances, the average American diet contains more than enough of these nutrients for daily activity.

Vitamins: The only vitamin that the body can produce is vitamin D. All other vitamins must be supplied by the diet. There are 13 known vitamins that fall into two classifications:

- Water Soluble
- Fat Soluble

The solubility of the vitamins must be kept in mind. The B-complex vitamins are water soluble while vitamins A,D,E and K are fat soluble. The ingestion of water soluble vitamins can usually be without consequence because they are eventually excreted in the urine. However, the fat soluble vitamins can potentially accumulate in the body leading to adverse consequences. Presently there are not much data supporting the use of vitamins to enhance performance beyond the daily recommended allowance. Most people consume more than enough vitamins each day by eating a variety of wholesome foods.

Minerals: Minerals are involved in many essential areas of bodily function. As is the case with vitamins, there is not data supporting the supplementation of minerals to improve performance, unless a state of deficiency exists. It is rare to have a mineral deficiency in an active person who is consuming a regular diet, with the exception of iron and calcium.

The dietary deficiency of iron is called anemia and may negatively affect performance. Iron is found in animal sources such as beef, lamb, or poultry. Plant sources such as peas, beans, and green vegetables are also sources of iron. Despite the apparent ease from which iron can be consumed in the diet anemia remains a problem especially for females.

Calcium is the most abundant mineral in the body and when combined with phosphorus forms bones and teeth. Calcium also exists in an ionized form, which is important in muscle function. Chronic calcium deficiency becomes prevalent later in life as osteoporosis and thin weak bones. A calcium deficiency can sometimes be found in young females who have poor eating habits.

Fluid and Electrolyte Balance: Proper hydration is critical. Dehydration becomes a bigger problem when physical training is involved. When you are thirsty, it is estimated you have already lost 1-2% of you bodyweight through dehydration. At this level it is estimated that athletic performance can decrease by 10-20%. Dehydration has also been shown to decrease peak rate of oxygen consumption during exercise at steady state work loads (VO_2 Max). At a minimum you should consume:

- 16oz 2 hrs prior to exercise
- 8-16oz 15 min prior to exercise
- Approx. 8oz every 15 minutes during exercise
- 20oz per pound of weight lost after exercise

As a general rule, your goal should be to match fluid intake with fluid loss as closely as possible. Intake of sodium and other electrolytes must be considered as electrolyte balance plays a key role in hydration status. Also, the addition of electrolytes usually makes fluids more palpable.

When replacing electrolytes, many people question how much electrolyte and potassium should be replacement beverages.

Units	Sodium	Potassium
mg/8 oz	165	46
mg/L	690	195
mEq/8 oz	7.2	1.2

Common Fluid Replacers

Drink	Calories per 8 oz	Potassium (mg) per 8 oz	Sodium (mg) per 8 oz
Gatorade	50	25	110
Coke	95	0	8
Pepsi	100	8	6
Orange Juice	110	475	2
Apple Juice	115	300	5
Cranberry Juice	150	60	10
Grape juice	155	335	5
Cranapple	175	70	5

Warning signs of dehydration can be subtle. Usually if you are thirsty, you are already dehydrated. Other earlier signs of dehydration are flushed skin, difficulty concentrating, loss of muscular endurance, cotton-mouth, headache, weakness, shortness of breath, indistinct speech, nausea/dry heaves, and dark urine. More ominous signs of dehydration include shriveled or swollen tongue, muscle spasms, delirium, sunken eyes, dim vision, inability to swallow, inability or painful urination, numb/cracked skin, stiffened eyelids, and deafness.

When monitoring fluid loss, look at urine color and odor. If you are hydrated properly, urine will be clear or pale yellow. When you need water, urine is dark yellow or brown. During training, learn your personal sweat rate: weigh yourself naked before and after a workout during which you consume no fluid. For each one pound of sweat lost, rehydrate with at least 16 ounces of fluid. For example, if two pounds are lost (32 oz) during exercise your target intake during your workout should be around 32 oz. A simpler way is to drink two cups of water for every pound you lose during activity.

What to look for in beverages:

- Should taste good
- Cause no gastric discomfort
- Rapidly absorbable
- Contain sodium and potassium

Special Environmental Conditions:

Hot and humid environments: The risks of dehydration and heat injury increase dramatically in hot, humid environments. Therefore, if you are doing your workout outdoors in the summer (or in a hot gym any time during the year), you need to be aware. When ambient temperature exceeds body temperature, heat cannot be dissipated by radiation. When relative humidity is high, the potential to dissipate heat by evaporation of sweat is substantially reduced. For example, at a relative humidity of 100%, evaporation of sweat does not occur. In humid environments, sweat drips from the body, leading to nonfunctional fluid loss. When temperature and humidity are both high, there is a higher risk of heat illness.

Cold environments: Although the risk of dehydration is greater in hot environments, dehydration is not uncommon in cool or cold weather. Your body's fluid loss through expiration is accelerated in cold dry environments. You also may not be aware of the sweat loss that may be high if insulated clothing is worn during intense exercise. In addition, people usually tend to have lower rates of fluid ingestion in cold environments.

Some examples to put it all in perspective:

If I am training for general health and fitness, how much energy nutrients (carbohydrates (CHO), protein (PRO), fat) should I consume per day?

Body Weight	50 kg	60 kg	70 kg	80 kg	90 kg	100 kg
CHO	240-320 g	320-460 g	340-500 g	460-540 g	480-580 g	520-640 g
PRO	45-60 g	55-95 g	65-100 g	65-120 g	75-130 g	80-130 g
FAT	15-30 g	20-40 g	20-40 g	25-50 g	25-50 g	30-60 g
Total kcals	1400-1700 kcals	1800-2100 kcals	1800-2400 kcals	2100-2700 kcals	2200-3100 kcals	2500-3500 kcals

If I am a recreational athlete, how much energy nutrients (carbohydrates (CHO), protein (PRO), fat) should I consume per day?

Body Weight	50 kg	60 kg	70 kg	80 kg	90 kg	100 kg
CHO	300-400 g	400-500 g	500-600 g	520-640 g	580-700 g	600-800 g
PRO	60-90 g	70-100 g	90-120 g	90-120 g	100-130 g	105-140 g
FAT	20-35 g	20-40 g	25-45 g	30-45 g	30-50 g	30-50 g
Total kcals	1700-1900 kcals	2000-2300 kcals	2300-2900 kcals	2600-3400 kcals	2900-3900 kcals	3000-4200 kcals

If I am a well-trained or elite athlete, how much energy nutrients (carbohydrates (CHO), protein (PRO), fat) should I consume per day?

Body Weight	50 kg	60 kg	70 kg	80 kg	90 kg	100 kg
CHO	460-500 g	520-600 g	580-700 g	640-800 g	720-900 g	800-1000 g
PRO	75-100 g	90-120 g	105-140 g	120-160 g	135-180 g	150-200 g
FAT	25-50 g	30-60 g	35-70 g	40-80 g	45-80 g	50-80 g
Total kcals	2100-2300 kcals	2600-2900 kcals	3000-3600 kcals	3400-4300 kcals	3800-5000 kcals	4200-5700 kcals

If you are eating around your workout program, keep in mind that carbohydrates and fluid before, during, and after exercise directly impact performance.

The previous sections were base theory and guidelines on proper nutrition and hydration. The ensuing sections are designed to provide specific examples and amounts in further detail on nutrition.

Nutrional Strategy:

Snacks before exercise: These snacks should:

- Contain relatively low amounts of fat and fiber, both of which delay stomach emptying.
- Provide sufficient fluid to maintain hydration.
- Provide adequate level of carbohydrates to maximize blood glucose maintenance.

Snacks during exercise: For workouts lasting less than 1 hour, snacks should be in the form of hydration to replace fluid losses. If a workout is longer than 1 hour, snacks should also provide carbohydrates (approximately 30-60 g/hour) for blood glucose level maintenance.

Snacks after exercise: These snacks should:

- Provide adequate energy and carbohydrates to replace muscle glycogen and to ensure rapid recovery.
    - If an athlete is glycogen-depleted, a carbohydrate intake of:
        - 1.5 grams per kilogram body weight during the first 30 minutes after exercise and again every 2 hours for 4-6 hours will be adequate to replace glycogen stores.
    - The best foods to eat after exercise are carbohydrates with a moderate to high glycemic index in the first half hour after exercise, followed by foods high in carbohydrate, with a low glycemic index.

Carbohydrates and Performance: Carbohydrates can serve to boost or increase performance. The question is: how much carbohydrate do you need and when?

- At exercise levels greater than 70% MHR aerobic capacity is fueled primarily by muscle glycogen and blood glucose.
- At exercise levels between 40-60% fat and carbohydrate are used in equal proportions.
- Fats contribute more to long durations of exercise.

Timing:

- Carbohydrates should be consumed 1 hour prior to activity.
- During activities lasting longer than 1 hour, carbohydrates should be consumed.
- After activity carbohydrates should be taken in three doses.
    - Within the first 30 minutes of the cessation of activity
    - Approximately two hours after activity
    - At or around four hours after activity

How Much:

- 1 hour prior to activity carbohydrate consumption is recommended at 1 gram per kilogram body weight.
- During activities that last longer than 1 hour 30-60g/hr should be ingested gradually in small increments and not as one large bolus. A bolus of food can lead to stomach upset. The body is

focusing blood flow and energy to the muscles and does not tolerate more than a small amount of food in the stomach at one time.

- After an activity, the carbohydrate ingested should be 1.5 grams per kilogram body weight. This maintains, over several hours, a constant supply of glucose to the recovering muscles and organs.

Carbohydrates before, during, and after a workout:

Body Weight	50 kg	60 kg	70 kg	80 kg	90 kg	100 kg
1 hr prior (1g/kg)	50 g	60 g	70 g	80 g	90 g	100 g
During	30-60 g/hr	30-60 g/hr	30-60 g/hr	30-60 g/hr	30-60 g/hr	30-60 g/hr
30 min after (1.5g/kg)	75 g	90 g	105 g	120 g	135 g	150 g
2 hr after (1.5g/kg)	75 g	90 g	105 g	120 g	135 g	150 g
4 hr after (1.5g/kg)	75 g	90 g	105 g	120 g	135 g	150 g

How much carbohydrate do I need?

Before workout/race: ~100 grams of carbohydrates (with a little protein and a little fat).
Eat 3-4 hours before the start time: research shows this will give you maximum benefits due to complete absorption.

Example meal #1:

- Two 6-inch whole wheat pancakes (45g)
- Spread with 3 teaspoons jam (14g)
- 1 cup sports drink (15g)
- Energy bar (45g)

119 grams carbohydrate total

Example meal #2:

- 1 cup cream of wheat (30g)
- Topped with 2 tablespoons honey (30g)
- One sliced banana-8 oz (30g),

90 grams carbohydrates total

Example meal #3:

- One whole wheat toasted bagel-4oz (60g)
- Spread with 2 tablespoons jam (27g)
- Liquid meal replacement such as Ensure or Boost (41g)

128 grams carbohydrates total

More examples of high carbohydrate, low-fat pre-workout meals

- Breakfast cereal + low-fat milk + fresh/canned fruit
- Muffins + jam/honey
- Pancakes + syrup
- Toast + baked beans (note this is a high-fiber choice) or spaghetti
- Creamed rice (made with low-fat milk)
- Rolls or sandwiches with banana filling
- Fruit salad + low-fat fruit yogurt
- Pasta with tomato or low-fat sauce
- Baked potatoes with low-fat filling
- Sports bars or cereal bars & sports drink
- Fruit smoothie (low-fat milk + fruit + low-fat yogurt/ ice cream)
- Liquid meal supplement

During the workout/race:
30-60 grams every hour.
Limited by gastrointestinal transit and absorption.

- All: 30 grams every ½ hour
- Sports drinks: approx 15 g carb/cup (8 oz.)
- Other options:
    - Sports gels (22g)
    - Energy bars (20-50g)
    - Consume these with 8 oz of water, not sports drink, to aid in absorption
    - No fiber, and limit protein and fat: these slow digestion and will make the much-needed carbohydrates inaccessible to you

After the workout/race
First 30 minutes:

- Bagels-4 oz (60g)
- Orange juice-8 oz (30g)
- Dried fruit 2/3 cup (80g)

170 g carbohydrate total

- If you are not hungry between events or right after exercise, then juices or sports drinks, which contain a lot of carbohydrates, will do the trick, as well as quench your thirst.

2 hrs after event:

- Meat or fish, wheat pasta 2 cups (60g)
- Beans 1 cup (30g)
- Whole grain bread (15g)
- Vegetables 2 cups (20g)

125 g carbohydrate total

More carbohydrate-rich foods

- Applesauce (1 cup) 60 g
- Banana (1) 27 g
- Cereal (1 cup) 24 g
- Corn (1 cup) 42 g
- Fig bars (4 cookies) 42 g
- Gatorade® (1 cup) 11 g
- Orange juice (1 cup) 26 g
- Pear (1) 25 g
- Potato (1 large) 50 g
- Raisins (2/3 cup) 79 g
- Rice (1 cup) 50 g

Carbohydrate Loading: (packing more glycogen in muscles and the liver): The most important fuel for muscle activity is carbohydrate. In the 1960s an idea came forth that increasing the carbohydrates ingested in the days prior to activity could increased the stored glycogen in the liver and muscles. This increased glycogen stores could result in more fuel for activity. This has repeatedly been shown to be effective for events lasting longer than 1 hour. However, in shorter events and workouts lasting less than 1 hour it has shown little, if any, benefit.

Supplements: As mentioned earlier, a well-balanced diet is all that is needed. However, there is a multi-billion dollar a year industry that is pushing dietary supplements. Dietary supplements include vitamins, minerals, botanicals, sports nutrition supplements, weight management products, and specialty supplements. Many of these commercially available products are designed as supplements, not as replacements for a well-balanced diet and a healthy lifestyle. In 1986 the dietary supplement industry was a $3 billion a year industry and by 2004 those sales increased to over $20 billion. The FDA lists 29,000 dietary supplements on the market today and estimates over 150 million Americans take one or more dietary supplement. Probably you or someone close to you has taken or currently takes some form of dietary supplement.

In 1994 the Dietary Supplements Health and Education Act (DSHEA) was signed recognizing that consumers believed dietary supplements to be safe and may confer health benefits. The U.S. Congress expanded on the DSHEA to include substances such as: ginseng, garlic, fish oils, psyllium, and enzymes. It is unfortunate that DSHEA has expanded the types of products that can be sold and increased the misinformation to consumers. The majority of diets are marketed without adequate research. Therefore, you should always use caution before starting any supplements. The FDA (Food and Drug Administration) does not regulate any of the commercially available products unless there are complaints. In addition, under DSHEA, dietary supplements do not have to pass pre-market safety evaluations nor are manufacturers required to demonstrate safety or effectiveness of their product. Therefore, the companies that produce the dietary supplements are able to market any claim they want. Consumers must be aware that supplements may not produce the advertised results and may even be harmful. A recent example of how a diets may be harmful are the deaths related to the appetite suppressant ephedra, that was removed from the market in 2004.

Most nutritional needs are met by a balanced diet, which comes at a more reasonable price than expensive supplements. Despite the seemingly unregulated market that dietary supplement deal in, certain information is required:

- Statement of identity (e.g. choline bitartrate)

- Net quantity of contents (e.g. 60 capsules)
- Structure function claim (e.g. what system of the body is affected and how this effect is accomplished.
- The statement: "This dietary supplement has not been evaluated by the Food and Drug Administration. This product is not intended to treat, cure, or prevent any disease".
- Directions for use (e.g. take one capsule daily)
- Supplement Facts panel (e.g. lists serving size, amount, and active ingredient)
- Other ingredients in descending order of predominance and by common name or proprietary blend
- Name and place of business manufacturer, packer, or distributor

Finally, it should be mentioned that some dietary supplements have been found to not contain what is printed on their labels. The supplement may contain none, little, or more of what is listed on the bottle contents.

Caffeine: Caffeine is often used as a stimulant in exercise. Some people feel that caffeine makes the effort seems easier. For others, caffeine can make people feel nervous, jittery or encourages multiple trips to the restroom. While caffeine has been shown to have a performance enhancing effect, it can also be dehydrating. It is a drug that is limited by the Olympic Committee.

Beer: Beer is a poor source of carbohydrates, electrolytes, and fluid before, during, or after exercise. The calories from beer are only 1/3 carbohydrate on average and light beer contains even fewer carbohydrates. Alcohol has a diuretic effect that contributes to increased fluid losses. If alcohol is going to be consumed it should be consumed after 2-3 cups of water and after having something to eat and used for its social value rather than use as a thirst quencher or fluid replacement.

Nutrition and Weight Loss: There are numerous weight loss and diet books, plans, and clubs in America that can overwhelm the average consumer in volume alone. Many times you might not know which direction to proceed or who to believe. The proliferation of fad diets has exploded in the last 20 years including the South Beach Diet, Atkins Diet, Scarsdale Diet, Russian Air Force Diet, and grapefruit diet to name only a few. Many of the authors of weight loss and diet books base their diets on anecdotal evidence, case studies, and vivid imaginations. Unfortunately some poorly conceived diets have resulted in deaths.

Weight is a variable that is constantly in a state of flux. Instead of weight loss, an alternative goal might be a refined physique, or a specific size of pants or shirt which you wish to fit into. Again, let how your clothes are fitting instead of your actual weight in pounds or kilograms define your goals with nutrition. If you absolutely demand to continue using a scale and monitoring weight, be certain you weigh yourself at the same time everyday, preferably first thing in the morning. Be aware that many factors, in particular hydration status, can greatly affect weight.

If you do begin a diet or diet plan choose one that focuses on changing individual behaviors. These should include long term changes in activities and caloric consumption. Short term fad diets that promote rapid weight loss are often useless and can even be harmful. The very rapid or accelerated weight losses claimed by some diets are produced by temporarily depletion of body of water. The depletion of body water can cause electrolyte imbalances, dehydration, and life-threatening irregular heart beats.

The best way to accomplish weight loss is by moderate changes in dietary behaviors and exercise patterns that can be sustained over the long term. The only reasonable diets on the market for weight loss should emphasize expending more energy through an increase in physical activity and ingesting fewer calories than you expend. The best diets are ones that effectively combine the two into a program that you can adopt and develop more beneficial eating and exercising behaviors. A well-planned diet will result in a loss of about 1 pound a week. When it comes to weight loss, Thomas Jefferson probably said it best:

"We seldom regret having eaten too little." – Thomas Jefferson

Final Thoughts on Nutrition: Regardless of athletic level of ability, each person should make eating an integral part of their training program and not just an afterthought. By practicing fueling before, during, and after exercise, the intestinal tract will learn how to manage food while exercising. This means more comfort and better performance. Everyone must learn how to manage their own body's nutrient requirements. Have fun by experimenting with different foods and fluids to determine what foods settle best. Gatorade or iced tea with honey? Energy bars or gummy bears? Dried fruit or gels?

Carbohydrate calories before exercise can enhance stamina and endurance. Some people believe that commercial sport foods are better than natural foods. For training, develop a menu of tried-and-true foods that digest well and taste good to you. This food may be one of the more enjoyable parts of the exercise experience, so choose wisely. Think about variety. Also, consider your healthy snacks following your workout to tide you over before a meal and replace glycogen losses.

You might also enjoy scheduling time to food shop. Set aside time to think about what to eat that day, so you can optimize you daily food intake. All too often, in the midst of juggling work, family, friends, sleep, and training, athletes find no time to plan meals and shop or obtain a well balanced sports diet. The result: another donut for breakfast, cookie for lunch, vending machine snack, and a fast 'n' fatty meal that fills the stomach but leaves muscles poorly fueled. Muscles need carbohydrates for fuel: oatmeal, granola, bagels, fruit, juice, hearty breads, and pasta. The goal is to eat carbohydrates evenly throughout the day. This is opposed to skimping on meals by day then gorging on treats at night. By having breakfast, a mid-morning snack, lunch, an afternoon snack, and dinner, one will have steady energy all day and avoid lags. Make time to develop an eating strategy that fits your training schedule.

A good resource when finding what types of food you should be eating comes from the U.S. Department of Agriculture's Food Pyramid and Dietary Guidelines. Here you can find recommendations for the proportions of foods that should be included in a healthy diet. Grains, vegetables, and fruits have the highest recommended number of servings and are excellent nutrient-rich sources of carbohydrates.

Recommendations for Further Reading:

1. *A Guide to Understanding Dietary Supplement*
   by Shawn M. Talbott, 713 pages, Publisher: Haworth Press (January, 2003), ISBN: 0789014564
2. *Dietary Supplements: Toxicology and Clinical Pharmacology*
   by Melanie Johns Cupp, Timothy S. Tracy, 450 pages, Publisher: Humana Press (January, 2003), ISBN: 158829014X
3. *Nancy Clark's Sports Nutrition Guidebook*
   by Nancy Clark, 416 pages, Publisher: Human Kinetics Publishers; 3rd ed (August, 2003), ISBN: 073604602X
4. *Nutrition for Serious Athletes*
   by Dan Benardot, 337 pages, Publisher: Human Kinetics Publishers (November, 1999), ISBN: 0880118334
5. *Sports Nutrition for Endurance Athletes*
   by Monique Ryan, 352 pages, Publisher: VeloPress (October, 2002), ISBN: 1931382158
6. *Sports Nutrition Guide: Minerals, Vitamins & Antioxidants for Athletes*
   by Michael Colgan, 298 pages, Publisher: Apple Publishing Company (WA) (March, 2002), ISBN: 0969527284

7. *The G.I. Handbook : How the Glycemic Index Works*
   by Barbara Ravage, 192 pages, Publisher: Barrons Educational Series (May 2, 2005), ISBN: 0764131605

8. *The Health Professional's Guide to Popular Dietary Supplements*
   by Allison Sarubin, 452 pages, Publisher: American Dietetic Association (2000), ISBN: 0880911808

9. *The New Glucose Revolution Complete Guide to Glycemic Index Values*
   by Jennie Brand-Miller, Kaye Foster-Powell, Susanna Holt, Johanna Burani, 144 pages, Publisher: Marlowe & Company (August 21, 2003), ISBN: 1569244782

10. *The New Glucose Revolution Shoppers' Guide to GI Values 2006 : The Authoritative Source of Glycemic Index Values for More than 500 Foods*
    by Dr. Jennie Brand-Miller, Kaye Foster-Powell, 192 pages, Publisher: Marlowe & Company (January 9, 2006), ISBN: 1569243298

11. *Training Nutrition: The Diet and Nutrition Guide for Peak Performance*
    by Ed Burke, Jacqueline R. Berning, 164 pages, Publisher: Cooper Pub Group (September 1, 1995), ISBN: 1884125220

12. United States Department of Agriculture. Food Guide Pyramid. Available online at: http://www.mypyramid.gov/

Not all those who know their minds know their hearts as well.
- Francois

Heart Rate: Heart rate is a term used to describe the frequency of the cardiac cycle. Usually it is calculated as the number of contractions (heart beats) of the heart in one minute and expressed as "beats per minute" (bpm). When resting, the adult human heart beats at about 70 bpm, but this rate varies between people. However, the reference range is nominally between 60 bpm (if less termed bradycardia) and 100 bpm (if greater, termed tachycardia). Resting heart rates can be significantly lower in athletes, and significantly higher in the obese.

The body can increase the heart rate in response to a wide variety of conditions in order to increase the cardiac output (the amount of blood ejected by the heart per unit time). Exercise or other stress causes a normal person's heart rate to increase above the resting heart rate.

The pulse is the most straightforward way of measuring the heart rate, but it can be deceptive when some strokes do not lead to much cardiac output. In these cases (as happens in some arrhythmias), the heart rate can be (much) higher than the pulse.

Choosing A Heart Rate Monitor: You can purchase a heart rate monitor (HRM) to measure accurately your heart rate during workouts for not much more than a regular sports wristwatch (<$50). Today, heart rate monitors are easier to use than they used to be. The most difficult task is picking the right model for you, given the many models on the market with the variety of functions.

Most heart rate monitors have two major pieces. A chest strap with monitor detects electrical activity and identifies each heart beat. This information is transmitted to a receiver, typically a wristwatch. The basic technology is similar regardless of make or model and there is little variability in device accuracy.

Basic models display heart rate alone. Additional functions available include stopwatch, countdown timer, splits/intervals, data recall, programmable heart rate zones, and at the high end: computer download ability and global positioning system (GPS). Functions such as countdown timer, splits/intervals, programmable heart rate zones and stopwatch you might find useful during MAX the MIN workouts. They allow you to accurately start and stop interval sessions, guide workout effort, gauge daily effort, and record training data for future analysis.

At a minimum most people select a heart rate monitor that also has a stopwatch facility, to save wearing two watches. Knowing exactly what you want your heart rate to be allows you to program heart rate ranges, with an upper and a lower limit. If you go too hard or too easy, the alarm will beep until you get back into your 'zone'.

One final aspect you should consider is the battery. With some models you can change the battery yourself, and others require you to send the whole monitor back to the manufacturer, which costs more and leaves you without your monitor for a while. However, your heart rate monitor is only as valuable as your ability to use it.

Measuring Heart Rate: Heart rate is commonly measured during active training and used as a guide to structure workouts and monitor physical effort. To use as a guide for training, heart rates are measured at complete rest and maximal effort. Resting heart rate (RHR) is the number of times your heart beats in one minute while at complete rest. The best way to measure your RHR is when you first wake up in the morning and before you get out of bed. Feel your pulse at your neck, count your pulse for 15 seconds and multiply by four. It is best to do this for five days and then average the results. RHR increases with age, illness, temperature, dehydration, certain medications, and higher altitudes. One sign of over-training is an elevated RHR. By becoming aware of your RHR you can more closely become in-tune with how your body is reacting to different stimuli. You should know that your RHR will decrease significantly after several weeks of an aerobic based workout program like MAX the MIN. After several months of regular physical exercise it would not be unusual for your RHR to be as low as 40-55 beats per minute (BPM). You may also notice that your heart rate following exercise will also be lower. A lower RHR and a lower heart rate after exercise indicate that your heart is working more efficiently.

Your maximum heart rate (MHR) is the fastest your heart is capable of beating in one minute at maximal effort. Unlike RHR, MHR does not typically show as drastic a decrease after several months of exercise. The average decrease in MHR after several months of aerobic exercise is approximately 3 bpm. Many eighteen to thirty year old individuals may have maximum heart rates at or exceeding 200 bpm. MHR decreases with age after the age of thirty, but some research seems to indicate that the gradual decrease with age is lessened with improved fitness. Once you know your MHR you will have an objective measure to the level of effort you are exerting. Adjusting this level of effort will allow for you to fine-tune your individual workout and training program, thereby increasing the effectiveness (e.g. efficiency) of time spent exercising. Measuring your own MHR is the most accurate way of determining your individual MHR. You may have it clinically tested (usually by treadmill stress testing) by a physician or exercise physiologist. You can also measure it in field conditions supervised by an experienced coach. If you are over the age of 35, overweight, have been sedentary for several years, or have a history of heart disease in your family, clinical testing is recommended. A final option is to measure you own maximum heart rate. Sports science laboratories often use a graded treadmill run to establish maximum heart rate. The speed of the treadmill is gradually increased until you can no longer keep up, and your heart rate at this point is assumed to be your maximum heart rate. Recent findings have suggested that a combination of short runs will give you higher readings than the traditional gradually increasing speed of the treadmill. To determine your MHR for strength and aerobic training program like MAX the MIN the following workout is recommended.

- After a proper warm up, do as many pullups as you can, immediately followed by the maximum pushups you can do in 1 minute followed by the maximum situps you can do in 1 minute. Rest two or three minutes of easy jogging, and then repeat your 3 exercise maximal effort.
- During the second effort you should get a higher maximum heart rate value than the first. Continue to use your monitor to take readings throughout it, as your heart rate may peak before the end.
- Shorter, faster bursts of less than three minutes don't appear to work, as the muscles then become exhausted before the cardio-respiratory system.

Needless to say, you should be in good physical health before you do any intensive exercise, let alone exercising to your body's upper limits. If you are in any doubt at all, get a medical check-up.

Target Heart Rate (THR): Target Heart Rate also know as "Training Heart Rate", is the range of heart rate which has been determined to give your cardiovascular system the max benefit from a workout. This range has several variables including:

- Physical condition

- Age
- Previous training

There are two common ways to calculate your THR. In both calculations the intensity is expressed as a percentage measured between 50-85%.

Standard Method:

The standard method for calculating THR is:
$$THR = MHR \times \%Intensity$$

Example for someone with a MHR of 180:
50% Intensity: $180 \times 0.50 = 90$ bpm
85% Intensity: $180 \times 0.85 = 153$ bpm

Karvonen Method:

The Karvonen formula for calculating THR is as follows:

Target Heart Rate (THR) = (MHR – RHR) × %Intensity) + RHR

Example for someone with a MHR of 180 and a RHR of 70:
50% intensity: $((180 - 70) \times 0.50) + 70 = 125$ bpm
85% intensity: $((180 - 70) \times 0.85) + 70 = 163$ bpm

Heart Rate Reserve (HRR): HRR is a term used to describe the difference between a person's RHR, and MHR. Some methods of measurement of exercise intensity measure percentage of HRR. Additionally, as a person becomes fit, as their RHR will drop, the HRR will increase.

- HRR = MHR - RHR

Heart Rate Variability (HRV): Heart rate variability (HRV) is the beat to beat variation of the heart rate. A healthy heart has large heart rate variability. What you will notice is that after several weeks of a cardiovascular workout like MAX the MIN your heart rate variability will increase (e.g. time for an elevated heart rate to return to normal). HRV can be used as an objective number to gauge fitness. The faster your heart rate returns to normal after stopping vigorous exercise indicates better fitness. A fit person's heart rate will return to a resting rate faster than an unfit person. A drop of 20 beats a minute is typical for a healthy person. Following exercise heart rate recovers in two phases:
- Phase I – seconds to two minutes after activity is stopped, heart rate decreases rapidly.
- Phase II – 2 to 10 minutes after activity is stopped, heart follows a slower decline returning to pre-exercise levels.

Exercise physiologists have divided the range between resting and maximal heart rate into several "zones." The heart rate increases in response to exercise have been linked to different levels of activity and energy systems. There are three energy systems in the body.

- **Adenosine triphosphate-creatine phosphate (ATP-CP/phosphagen) system:** Sustains all out effort for 5-8 seconds. During the MAX the MIN workout your first repetitions make utilize this energy system.

- **Anaerobic (lactic acid) System:** The breakdown of energy with oxygen is typically called anaerobic metabolism. Anaerobic metabolism provides a rapid very accessible, yet limited energy source for muscular activity. Generally speaking, anaerobic metabolism is used during sprinting, weight lifting, and jumping. It can sustain exercise for 60 seconds, and only glucose can be used for fuel, with lactic acid accumulation. During the MAXimize the MINimum you will spend some of your time in this training zone.

- **Aerobic:** The breakdown of energy using oxygen is referred to as aerobic metabolism. At rest or with minimal activity the energy source is typically fatty acids while with increasing demand glucose and its stored form glycogen become more important. Aerobic mechanisms supply most of the body's energy at any given time. Aerobic metabolism is used during endurance training that involves repetitive dynamic, rhythmic movements of the large muscles for a prolonged time. As length of exercise increases the amount of aerobically produced energy increases. Some examples of primarily aerobic activities are distance swimming, distance cycling, distance running, and cross-country skiing.

Heart Rate Zones: Heart rate training zones are designed to match your desired training outcome to the right type of program. Training intensity, and therefore the training HR zone, should be higher for shorter events, and lower for longer endurance events. There are 4 training zones or heart rate ranges. Heart rate zones are arbitrary divisions and can differ from coach to coach. They are based on the increase in heart rate as the oxygen consumption of the exercising muscle increases, and the concept of the benefits of variable stress in developing the exercising muscle. As you move up the hierarchy of training zones, exercise intensity increases and there is a shift from the use of fat as an energy source for the muscle to carbohydrate. As the MHR is reached, there is a shift in the muscle cell towards anaerobic metabolism.

The Heart Rate Intensity Zones are divided as follows:

- Zone 1 60-70% of MHR
- Zone 2 71-80% of MHR
- Zone 3 81-85% of MHR
- Zone 4 >85% of MHR

If you always train at low heart rates, you will develop excellent endurance with no top strength. Conversely if you train hard most of the time, you'll never recover completely and chronic fatigue will poison your performance. The solution is to mix hard training with easy training in the proper proportions.

The best approach is to stay below 80% of maximum heart rate (zones 1 to 3) for the majority of your workout and then push above 80% when it's time to go hard to improve your high level performance. Train below 80% MHR with spikes into the 80-85% range early in the workout and spikes into the >85% range later in the workout as your muscles become fully warmed up. It has been determined that the optimal intensity for aerobic based training occurs between 60-80% MHR. Keeping your average heart rate between these two variables has shown the most favorable long-term adaptation and improvement in oxygen transport capacity. Little additional cardiorespiratory benefit has been seen at higher intensity training >80%MHR, but may give benefits by helping the heart pump an increased amount of blood with each beat.

Zone 1: *Light intensity (60 – 70% of MHR) "Fat Burn"*
Exercising at this intensity, you will notice your breathing is slightly labored, but, if you have a training partner, you can still talk quite freely. With practice, you will be able to continue exercising at this level for long periods. This range can be obtained through brisk walking, jogging, swimming and cycling. You will burn around 40% fat and 60% carbohydrate.

Zone 2: *Moderate intensity (71 – 80% of MHR)*
This zone will improve your cardiovascular and respiratory system and is the most efficient at increasing the size and strength of your heart. This is the preferred zone if you are training for an endurance event. You will still be able to talk to a training partner, but conversation may be a little more blunted and not as free. Calories burned are typically 30-40% from fat and 60-70% from carbohydrates. You goal in the MAX the MIN workout is to have the majority of your time spent in this zone.

Zone 3: *No Man's Land (81-85% of MHR)*
The "no man's land" or "mediocre middle" at 81-85% of MHR is too difficult to maintain and is not the most efficient zone for building endurance or strength. Early in your workout your exercises may spike into this zone, but if your heart rate is consistently in this zone take more rest to allow yourself to recover in the moderate intensity zone (71-80% MHR). Unfortunately, this is the zone that many untrained and uneducated people train.

Zone 4: *High intensity (above 85% of MHR)*
At this intensity, you don't want to talk to anybody. You are truly focused on your workout. Your body is extracting an increased proportion of its energy from carbohydrates stored within contracting muscles and elsewhere, since oxygen delivery alone is too slow to meet the needs of the contracting muscles. The greater the intensity, the shorter the time it can be maintained. Some examples of similar exercises that are spent in these zones include: running intervals, uphill cross-country skiing, and very intense swimming and cycling. Several times near the end of your workout of MAXimize the Minimum you will venture into this area. During this time you will be training your anaerobic system.

Recommendations for Further Reading:

1. *Precision Heart Rate Training*
   by Edmund Burke, 211 pages, Publisher: Human Kinetics Publishers (March, 1998), ISBN: 0880117702
2. *The High Performance Heart: Effective Training for Health, Fitness and Competition With the Heart Rate Monitor*
   by Philip Maffetone, Matthew Mantell, 160 pages, Publisher: Motorbooks International; 2nd/Rev/Up edition (September, 1994), ISBN: 0933201648

CHAPTER 7: What about when I'm Traveling?
(Modified workouts for those on the road)

Life is either a daring adventure or nothing.
-Helen Keller

Sometimes an individual cannot commit an hour to the routines described above. In that case, you should improvise your workout. First check to see if your hotel has a gym with a pullup bar, or perhaps the desk attendant knows of a school or park nearby that you can visit. If neither is available, look around the hotel room. Where can you tuck your toes to do situps? Is there 8 feet of open floor space for some pushups, V-ups, or maybe even some flutter kicks? Finally, find two chairs to do some pseudo dips. You will be amazed at how much you are still able to do (Again, MAX the MIN – you will be getting the maximum workout with the minimum equipment). After 30 minutes of exercise you will feel rejuvenated and glad you worked out.

Modified Workouts:

Beginner:

10x2 pullups
10x10 pushups
10x4 dips
10x10 situps
10x10 lunges

Total time: 30 minutes
Completed on 30 second time interval

Intermediate:

10x5 pullups
10x12 pushups
10x8 dips
10x12 situps
10x12 lunges

Total time: 30 minutes
Completed on 30 second time interval

Hard:

10x10 pullups
10x15 pushups
10x12 dips
10x15 situps
10x15 lunges

Total time: 30 minutes
Completed on 30 second time interval

When pull up and dip bars are not available, one can to the following:

Beginner:

10x10 pushups
10x10 situps
10x8 chair dips
10x8 lunges

Total time: 40 minutes
Completed on 1 minute time interval

Intermediate:

10x15 pushups
10x15 situps
10x12 chair dips
10x12 lunges

Total time: 40 minutes
Completed on 1 minute time interval

Hard:

10x25 pushups
10x25 situps
10x20 chair dips
10x20 lunges

Total time: 40 minutes
Completed on 1 minute time interval

The key here is to strive to maintain your fitness despite the changed surrounding and environment. You can do it. Now, Turn off that HBO movie and get down to business.

APPENDIX A: Weekly Schedules

As a guideline for structuring your routine, you might want to keep track of your work-outs.

Sample Weekly Schedule:

<u>Sunday</u>: :30 min   Total time*: :30 min

<u>Monday</u>: off   Total time*: 0

<u>Tuesday</u>: off   Total time*: 0

<u>Wednesday</u>: :30 min   Total time*: :30 min

<u>Thursday</u>: off   Total time*: 0

<u>Friday</u>: off   Total time*: 0

<u>Saturday</u>: :30 min   Total time*: :30 min

<u>Weekly Totals:</u>

Exercise 1:_____Interval:_____
Exercise 2:_____Interval:_____
Exercise 3:_____Interval:_____
Exercise 4:_____Interval:_____
Exercise 5:_____Interval:_____
Exercise 6:_____Interval:_____
Exercise 7:_____Interval:_____
Exercise 8:_____Interval:_____

You can estimate the amount of time you were in the following heart rate zones.
(60-70% MHR):_____
(70-80% MHR):_____
(85% + up):_____

Notes

_____
_____
_____
_____
_____
_____
_____
_____

Alternate Weekly Beginner:

Sunday: off   Total time*: 0

Monday: :30 min   Total time*: :30 min

Tuesday: off   Total time*: 0

Wednesday: :30 min Total time*: :30 min

Thursday: off   Total time*: 0

Friday: :30 min   Total time*: :30 min

Saturday: off   Total time*: 0

Weekly Totals:

Exercise 1:_____Interval:_____
Exercise 2:_____Interval:_____
Exercise 3:_____Interval:_____
Exercise 4:_____Interval:_____
Exercise 5:_____Interval:_____
Exercise 6:_____Interval:_____
Exercise 7:_____Interval:_____
Exercise 8:_____Interval:_____

You can estimate the amount of time you were in the following heart rate zones.
(60-70% MHR):_____
(70-80% MHR):_____
(85% + up):_____

Notes

_____
_____
_____
_____
_____
_____
_____
     _____

APPENDIX B: Daily Training Log
MAXimize the MINimum
Daily Workout Schedule
Date:_____

Day:_____of_____

Planned Workout

Exercise	Reps	Interval

Actual Workout

Exercise	Reps	Interval

Planned Total Time: _____

Actual Total Time: _____

Notes

_____
_____
_____
_____
_____
_____

Plan

Exercise: Continue / Change (New Exercise:_____)

Reps: Decrease / Maintain / Increase

Interval: Decrease / Maintain / Increase

MAXimize the MINimum
Daily Nutrition Schedule

Date: _____

Day:_____of_____

Planned Menu

	Time	Food	Fluid Type	fl oz
Meal #1				
Snack #1				
Meal #2				
Snack #2				
Meal #3				
Snack #3				

Actual Menu

	Time	Food	Fluid Type	fl oz
Meal #1				
Snack #1				
Meal #2				
Snack #2				
Meal #3				
Snack #3				

Planned Totals:

Grains (ounce equivalents):_____

Vegetables (cups):_____

Fruits (cups):_____

Milk (cups):_____

Meat & Beans (ounce equivalents):_____

Oils & Discretionary Calories (teaspoons):_____

Fluid Intake (ounces):_____

Actual Totals:

Grains (ounce equivalents):_____

Vegetables (cups):_____

Fruits (cups):_____

Milk (cups):_____

Meat & Beans (ounce equivalents):_____

Oils & Discretionary Calories (teaspoons):_____

Fluid Intake (ounces):_____

Notes

_____

_____

I was hungry today: Yes / No   I was thirsty today: Yes / No

My energy level was: Low / Average / High

Increase/Decrease: Fluids / Grains / Vegetables / Fruits / Milk / Meat&Beans

MAXimize the MINimum
Monthly Schedule
Dates:_____
Weeks 1-12
Week 1 – Hard (Experiment with the MAX the MIN and find the exercises you enjoy)
Week 2 – Hard (increase reps and/or decrease interval by 10% or less)
Week 3 – Hard (increase reps and/or decrease interval by 10% or less)
Week 4 – Rest (decrease reps and/or decrease interval by 40%)
Week 5 – Hard (increase reps and/or decrease interval by 10% or less)
Week 6 – Hard (increase reps and/or decrease interval by 10% or less)
Week 7 – Hard (Max week: One hard day/easy day followed by a workout of maximums)
Week 8 – Rest (decrease reps and/or decrease interval by 40%)
Week 9 – Hard (Redefine your workout based on results of Week 7)
Week 10 – Hard (increase reps and/or decrease interval by 10% or less)
Week 11 – Hard (Max week: One hard day/easy day followed by a workout of maximums)
Week 12 – Rest (decrease reps and/or decrease interval by 40%)

Plan

What exercises do you like/dislike:_____
Which exercises are challenging/not challenging
enough:_____
Are you satisfied with the results: Yes   /   No
Comments:_____
Weeks 13-24
Week 13 – Hard (Experiment with the MAX the MIN Workout and vary your exercises)
Week 14 – Hard (increase reps and/or decrease interval by 10% or less)
Week 15 – Hard (increase reps and/or decrease interval by 10% or less)
Week 16 – Rest (decrease reps and/or decrease interval by 40%)
Week 17 – Hard (increase reps and/or decrease interval by 10% or less)
Week 18 – Hard (increase reps and/or decrease interval by 10% or less)
Week 19 – Hard (Max week: One hard day/easy day followed by a workout of maximums)
Week 20 – Rest (decrease reps and/or decrease interval by 40%)
Week 21 – Hard (Redefine your workout based on results of Week 7)
Week 22 – Hard (increase reps and/or decrease interval by 10% or less)
Week 23 – Hard (Max week: One hard day/easy day followed by a workout of maximums)
Week 24 – Rest (decrease reps and/or decrease interval by 40%)

Plan

What exercises do you like/dislike:_____
Which exercises are challenging/not challenging
enough:_____
Are you satisfied with the results: Yes   /   No
Comments:_____

REFERENCES

1. American College of Sports Medicine. (1990) The recommended quantity and quality of exercise for developing an maintaining cardiorespiratory and muscular fitness in healthy adults. Sports Med Bull 13(3):1-4.

2. Andrade, M., (2004) Dietary long-chain omega-3 fatty acids and anti-inflammatory action: potential application in the field of physical exercise. *Nutrition.* 20: 243.

3. Available online: http://www.cdc.gov/nccdphp/sgr/sgr.htm

4. Birrer, RB, O'Connor, FG, Sports Medicine for the Primary Care Physician, 3rd ed. Boca Raton, CRC Press, 2004.

5. Borenstein D. (1996) Epidemiology, etiology, diagnostic evaluation, and treatment of low back pain. *Curr Opin Rheumatol* Mar; 8(2): 124-9

6. Calle EE, Rodriguez C, Walker-Thurmond K, Thun MJ. (2003) Overweight, obesity, and mortality from cancer in a prospectively studied cohort of U.S. adults. *New England Journal of Medicine* 348(17):1625–1638.

7. Campbell, W., Crim, M., Young, V. and Evans, W. (1994). Increased energy requirements and changes in body composition with resistance training in older adults. *American Journal of Clinical Nutrition*, 60: 167-175.

8. Clark, D. O., Stump, T. E., Damush, T. M. (2003). Outcomes of an Exercise Program for Older Women Recruited through Primary Care. *J Aging Health* 15: 567-585

9. Cornelissen, V. A., Fagard, R. H. (2005). Effects of Endurance Training on Blood Pressure, Blood Pressure-Regulating Mechanisms, and Cardiovascular Risk Factors. *Hypertension* 46: 667-675

10. Dehn, MM, Mullins, CB, (1977) Physiologic effects and importance of exercise in patients with coronary artery disease. *Cardiovasc Med* 2:365-387

11. Dietary Supplement Health and Education Act of 1994, Pub L No. 103.417.

12. Duncan, J. J., Farr, J. E., Upton, J., Hagan, R. D., Oglesby, M. E., & Blair, S. N. (1985). The effects of aerobic exercise on plasma catecholamines and blood pressure in patients with mild hypertension. *J American Medical Association* 254: 2609-2613

13. Evans, W. and Rosenberg, I. (1992). *Biomarkers*. New York: Simon and Schuster.

14. Flegal K.M., Carroll M.D., Ogden C.L., Johnson C.L.. (2002) Prevalence and trends in obesity among U.S. adults, 1999–2000. *J American Medical Association* 288(14):1723–1727.

15. Fontanarrosa, P.B., Rennie, D., DeAngelis, C.D., (2003) The Need for Regulation of Dietary Supplements—Lessons From Ephedra. (editorial). *JAMA,* 289:1568-1570.

16. Forbes, G. B. (1976). "The adult decline in lean body mass," *Human Biology*, 48: 161-73.

17. Foss, ML, Keteyian, SJ, Fox's Physiological Basis for Exercises and Sport, 6th ed. Boston, McGraw-Hill, 1998.

18. Friedenreich CM. (2001) Physical activity and cancer prevention: From observational to intervention research. *Cancer Epidemiology, Biomarkers and Prevention* 10(4):287–301.

19. Greenleaf, J. E., (1992) Problem: thirst, drinking behavior and involuntary dehydration. *Medicine and Science in Sports and Exercise*, 24:645-656

20. Harper, C.R., Jacobson, T.A., (2005) Usefulness of Omega-3 Fatty Acids and the Prevention of Coronary Heart Disease. *The American Journal of Cardiology.* 96: 1521-1529.

21. Huang Z, Hankinson SE, Cloditz GA, et al. (1997). Dual effects of weight and weight gain on breast cancer risk. *J American Medical Association* 278(17):1407–1411

22. Hultman E, Harris RC, Spriet LL: Work and exercise. *In* Shils ME, Olson JA, Shike M, et al (eds): Modern Nutrition in Health and Disease, 9th ed. Philadelphia, Lippincott Williams & Wilkins, 1999.

23. Keyes, A., Taylor, H. L. and Grande, F. (1973). "Basal Metabolism and Age of Adult Man," *Metabolism.* 22: 579-87.

24. Kokkinos, P.F., Narayan, P.N., Colleran, J.A., Pittaras, A., Notargiacomo, A., Reda, D., Papademetriou, V. (1995). Effects of Regular Exercise on Blood Pressure and Left Ventricular Hypertrophy in African-American Men with Severe Hypertension. *New England Journal of Medicine* 333: 1462-1467

25. Kremer JM, Lawrence DA, Jubiz W, DiGiacomo R, Rynes R, Bartholomew LE, et al. (1990) Dietary fish oil and olive oil supplementation in patients with rheumatoid arthritis. Clinical and immunologic effects. *Arthritis Rheum.* 33:810–20.

26. Cleland LG, French JK, Betts WH, Murphy GA, Elliott MJ. (1988) Clinical and biochemical effects of dietary fish oil supplements in rheumatoid arthritis. *J Rheumatol* 15:1471–5.

27. Lau CS, Morley KD, Belch JJ. (1993) Effects of fish oil supplementation on non-steroidal anti-inflammatory drug requirement in patients with mild rheumatoid arthritis—a double-blind placebo controlled study. *Br J Rheumatol* 32:982–9.

28. Martin, W.F., Armstrong, L.E., Rodriguez, N.R., (2005) Dietary protein intake and renal function. *Nutrition & Metabolism* 2:25.

29. Mensink RPM, Katan MB.(1990) Effect of dietary trans fatty acids on high-density and low-density lipoprotein cholesterol levels in healthy subjects. *N Engl J Med* 323:439–45.

30. National Heart, Lung, and Blood Institute. (1998). Clinical Guidelines on the Identification, Evaluation, and Treatment of Overweight and Obesity in Adults. *NIH Publication* No. 98–4083. Bethesda, MD.

31. Nieuwland, W, Berkhuysen, MA, Van Veldhuisen, DJ, Rispens, P, (2002) Individual assessment of intensity-level for exercise training in patients with coronary artery disease is necessary. *Int J Cardiology* 84(1):15-20

32. NIH (1993). The fifth report of the joint national committee on detection, evaluation, and treatment of high blood pressure. *Arch of Intern Med* 153: 154-183

33. Polednak AP. (2003) Trends in incidence rates for obesity-associated cancers in the U.S. *Cancer Detection and Prevention* 27(6):415–421.

34. Pollock, MI., Gettman LR, Milesis CA., et al: (1977) Effects of frequence and duration of training on attrition and incidence of injury. *Med Sci Sports* 9:31-36

35. Rakel D, Integrative Medicine, 1st ed. Philadelphia, W.B. Saunders Company, 2003.

36. Rakel R, Textbook of Family Practice, 6th ed. W. B. Saunders Company, 2002.

37. Robergs, RA, Landwehr, R, (2002) The Surprising History of the "HRmax=220-age" Equation. *J of Exercise Physiology Online* 5(2):1-10

38. Southhard, T.L., Pugh, J. W., (2004). Effect of Hydration State on Heart Rate Based Estimates of VO$_2$ Max. *J of Exercise Physiology Online*, 7:19-25

39. Strauss, RH, Strauss Sports Medicine, 2nd ed. Philadelphia, W.B. Saunders, 1991.

40. U.S. DEPARTMENT OF HEALTH AND HUMAN SERVICES
Centers for Disease Control and Prevention

National Center for Chronic Disease Prevention and Health Promotion
The President's Council on Physical Fitness and Sports

41. US Food and Drug Administration. Overview of dietary supplements. Available at: http://www.cfsan.fda.gov/ ~dms/ds-oview.html. Accessibility verified January 16, 2006.
42. US Food and Drug Administration. Overview of dietary supplements. Available at: http://www.cfsan.fda.gov/~dms/ds-ind.html. Accessibility verified January 16, 2006.
43. US Food and Drug Administration. Overview of dietary supplements. Available at: http://www.cfsan.fda.gov/~dms/hclaims.html. Accessibility verified January 16, 2006.
44. van den Brandt PA, Spiegelman D, Yuan SS, et al. (2000) Pooled analysis of prospective cohort studies on height, weight, and breast cancer risk. *American Journal of Epidemiology* 152(6):514–527.
45. Volker D, Fitzgerald P, Major G, Garg M. (2000) Efficacy of fish oil concentrate in the treatment of rheumatoid arthritis. *J Rheumatol* 27:2343–6.
46. Weir, M. R., Maibach, E. W., Bakris, G. L., Black, H. R., Chawla, P., Messerli, F. H., Neutel, J. M., Weber, M. A. (2000). Implications of a Health Lifestyle and Medication Analysis for Improving Hypertension Control. *Arch Intern Med* 160: 481-490

ABOUT THE AUTHORS

James Bales was born in eastern Colorado. He attended the United States Air Force Academy where he obtained his Bachelor of Science in biochemistry and learned the underlying physiologic processes of how the body works. While at the Air Force Academy he had the distinction of being named an All-American in both swimming and the triathlon. During this time, he also attended Navy Dive School, Airborne, Air Assault, and Combat Survival Training. A 2001 distinguished graduate from the Air Force Academy, Dr. Bales was the number one graduate in physical fitness in a class of 891, setting many school fitness records. Dr. Bales then attended Georgetown University School of Medicine where he graduated with honors in 2005 with a Medical Doctor degree. Despite the demands of medical school, he continued to compete in triathlons, and in 2004 turned professional in the sport. He attributes much of his success to the routines described in this text, which represent a culmination of what he had learned regarding physical fitness. While in medical school, Dr. Bales worked as the Head Endurance Trainer at Gold's Gym, Washington D.C., and personally coached and worked with numerous elite and professional athletes. Currently, Dr. Bales is commissioned as a captain in the U.S. Air Force and is completing his orthopaedic surgery residency at Wilford Hall Medical Center in San Antonio Texas where he is actively engaged in the training of Combat Control, Para Rescue, and Combat Survival students at Lackland Air Force Base.

Peter Andrews is a Professor in the Department of Biochemistry, Molecular and Cell Biology at the Georgetown University School of Medicine. Born in Takoma Park Maryland, Dr. Andrews received a Bachelor of Science degree from American University in Washington, D.C., a Master of Science from Georgetown University in Washington, D.C., and a Ph.D. from Tulane University in New Orleans, LA. Like Dr. Bales, Dr. Andrews excelled in physical fitness competitions and participated in many collegiate sports including wrestling (MVP), track and field, soccer, racquetball and volleyball. Dr. Andrews has author or co-authored over a hundred scientific articles over a wide range of biomedical topics and directed several major medical school courses at the Georgetown University School of Medicine. With the full-time demands of combined teaching and research associated with academia, Dr. Andrews recognized the physical and emotional benefits of the time efficient routines developed by Dr. Bales. It was from seeing the outstanding results of these routines that inspired the collaboration for this publication.